U.S. NAVY

U.S. MARINE CORPS

NTTP 4-02.2M

MCRP 4-11.1G

I0415652

PATIENT MOVEMENT

EDITION MAY 2007

DEPARTMENT OF THE NAVY
OFFICE OF THE CHIEF OF NAVAL OPERATIONS

DISTRIBUTION RESTRICTION:
APPROVED FOR PUBLIC RELEASE;
DISTRIBUTION IS UNLIMITED.

PRIMARY REVIEW AUTHORITY:
CHIEF, BUREAU OF MEDICINE
AND SURGERY

URGENT CHANGE/ERRATUM RECORD		
NUMBER	DATE	ENTERED BY

DEPARTMENT OF THE NAVY
OFFICE OF THE CHIEF OF NAVAL OPERATIONS AND
HEADQUARTERS, U.S. MARINE CORPS

MARINE CORPS DISTRIBUTION: PCN 144 000166 00

0411LP1066670

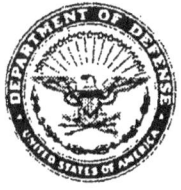

DEPARTMENT OF THE NAVY

BUREAU OF MEDICINE AND SURGERY
WASHINGTON, DC 20372-5300

March 2007

LETTER OF APPROVAL

1. NTTP 4-02.2M/MCRP 4-11.1G (MAY 2007), PATIENT MOVEMENT, is UNCLASSIFIED. Handle in accordance with the administrative procedures contained in NTTP 1-01.

2. NTTP 4-02.2M/MCRP 4-11.1G (MAY 2007) is effective upon receipt and supersedes NTTP 4-02.2, PATIENT MOVEMENT, dated April 2001. Destroy superseded material without report.

3. NTTP 4-02.2M/MCRP 4-11.1G (MAY 2007) addresses U.S. Navy and Marine Corps patient movement capabilities available to the operational commander. This publication prescribes tactics, techniques, and procedures for theater operations, mission planning, and training.

4. NTTP 4-02.2M/MCRP 4-11.1G (MAY 2007) is approved for public release; distribution is unlimited.

Approved

D. C. ARTHUR

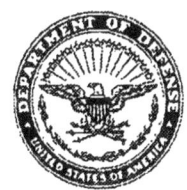

DEPARTMENT OF THE NAVY

NAVY WARFARE DEVELOPMENT COMMAND
NEWPORT, RI 02841-1207
MARINE CORPS COMBAT DEVELOPMENT COMMAND
QUANTICO, VA 22134-5001

May 2007

LETTER OF PROMULGATION

1. NTTP 4-02.2M/MCRP 4-11.1G (MAY 2007), PATIENT MOVEMENT, is UNCLASSIFIED. Handle in accordance with the administrative procedures contained in NTTP 1-01.

2. NTTP 4-02.2M/MCRP 4-11.1G (MAY 2007) is effective upon receipt and supersedes NTTP 4-02.2, PATIENT MOVEMENT, dated April 2001. Destroy superseded material without report.

3. NTTP 4-02.2M/MCRP 4-11.1G (MAY 2007) addresses U.S. Navy and Marine Corps patient movement capabilities available to the operational commander. This publication prescribes tactics, techniques, and procedures for theater operations, mission planning, and training.

4. NTTP 4-02.2M/MCRP 4-11.1G (MAY 2007) is approved for public release; distribution is unlimited.

BY DIRECTION OF THE COMMANDANT OF THE MARINE CORPS

JAMES F. AMOS
Lieutenant General, U.S. Marine Corps
Deputy Commandant for Combat Development and Integration

CARLTON B. JEWETT
Commander
Navy Warfare Development Command

May 2007

PUBLICATION NOTICE   ROUTING

1. NTTP 4-02.2M/MCRP 4-11.1G (MAY 2007), PATIENT MOVEMENT, is
   available in the Navy Warfare Library. It is effective upon receipt.

2. This publication addresses Navy and Marine Corps patient movement capabilities
   available to the operational commander; prescribes tactics, techniques, and
   procedures for theater operations; and describes mission planning and training.
   It is a complete revision of the previous publication and should be read in its
   entirety.

3. Summary. This publication is a reference for operational commanders, planners,
   and health service support personnel on Navy and Marine Corps patient movement
   operations. It summarizes tactics, techniques, and procedures and incorporates
   lessons learned from recent operations. Other users are unified, joint, and supported
   commanders and planners responsible for theater health service support.

Navy Warfare Library Custodian

Navy Warfare Library publications must be made
readily available to all users and other interested
personnel within the U.S. Navy.

Note to Navy Warfare Library Custodian

This notice should be duplicated for routing to cognizant personnel to keep them informed of changes to this
publication.

CONTENTS

CHAPTER 4 — NAVY PATIENT MOVEMENT OPERATIONS

CHAPTER 5 — MARINE CORPS PATIENT MOVEMENT OPERATIONS

MAY 2007

APPENDIX D — EXAMPLES OF STATUS BOARDS USED IN MEDICAL REGULATING

APPENDIX E — CASUALTY CATEGORIZATION AND PRIORITIZATION

APPENDIX F — AFLOAT AND SHIPBOARD MEDICAL EVACUATION CHECKLISTS

REFERENCES

LIST OF ACRONYMS AND ABBREVIATIONS

LIST OF ILLUSTRATIONS

PREFACE

NTTP 4-02.2M/MCRP 4-11.1G, PATIENT MOVEMENT (MAY 2007), addresses Navy and Marine Corps patient movement capabilities available to the operational commander and prescribes tactics, techniques, and procedures (TTPs) for theater operations, mission planning, and training. It is a complete revision of the previous publication and should be read in its entirety. This NTTP is not intended to prevent an officer who is exercising tactical command from initiating and issuing special instructions. Its primary purpose is to obtain basic uniformity while permitting the development and flexibility required by each tactical situation.

Report administrative discrepancies by letter, message, or e-mail to:

COMMANDER
NAVY WARFARE DEVELOPMENT COMMAND
ATTN: N5
686 CUSHING ROAD
NEWPORT RI 02841-1207

fleetpubs@nwdc.navy.mil

ORDERING DATA

Navy. Order printed copies of a publication using the Print on Demand (POD) system. A command may requisition a publication using standard military requisitioning and issue procedures (MILSTRIP) or the Naval Supply Systems Command (NAVSUP) website called the Naval Logistics Library (NLL) (www.nll.navsup.navy.mil). An approved requisition is forwarded to the specific Document Automation and Production Service (DAPS) site at which the publication's electronic file is officially stored. Currently, two copies are printed at no cost to the requester.

Marine Corps. A printed copy of a publication may be obtained from Marine Corps Logistics Base, Albany, GA 31704-5001, by following the instructions in MCBul 5600, *Marine Corps Doctrinal Publications Status*. An electronic copy may be obtained from the Marine Corps Combat Development Command (MCCDC), Doctrine World Wide Web home page, which is found at the following universal reference locator: https://www.doctrine.usmc.mil.

CHANGE RECOMMENDATIONS

Procedures for recommending changes are provided below.

WEB-BASED CHANGE RECOMMENDATIONS

Recommended changes to this publication may be submitted to the Navy Warfare Development Doctrine Discussion Group (DDG), accessible through the Navy Warfare Development Command (NWDC) website at: http://www.nwdc.navy.smil.mil/.

URGENT CHANGE RECOMMENDATIONS

When items for changes are considered urgent, send this information by message to the Primary Review Authority (PRA), info NWDC. Clearly identify and justify both the proposed change and its urgency. Information addressees should comment as appropriate. See accompanying sample for urgent change recommendation format on page 16.

ROUTINE CHANGE RECOMMENDATIONS

Navy. Submit routine recommended changes to this publication at any time by using the accompanying routine change recommendation letter format on page 17 and mailing it to the address below, or posting the recommendation on the NWDC Doctrine Discussion Group site.

COMMANDER
NAVY WARFARE DEVELOPMENT COMMAND
DOCTRINE DIRECTOR (N5)
686 CUSHING ROAD
NEWPORT RI 02841-1207

Marine Corps. Readers of this publication are encouraged to submit suggestions and changes through the Universal Need Statement (UNS) process. The UNS submission process is delineated in Marine Corps Order 3900.15A, *Marine Corps Expeditionary Force Development System,* which can be obtained from the Marine Corps Publications Electronic Library Online (universal reference locator: http://www.usmc.mil/directiv.nsf/web+orders). The UNS recommendation should include the following information:

- Location of change
    Publication number and title
    Current page number
    Paragraph number (if applicable)
    Line number
    Figure or table number (if applicable)

- Nature of change
    Addition/deletion of text
    Proposed new text

CHANGE BARS

Revised text is indicated by a black vertical line in the outside margin of the page, like the one printed next to this paragraph. The change bar indicates added or restated information. A change bar in the margin adjacent to the chapter number and title indicates a new or completely revised chapter.

WARNINGS, CAUTIONS, AND NOTES

The following definitions apply to warnings, cautions, and notes used in this manual:

WARNING

An operating procedure, practice, or condition that may result in injury or death if not carefully observed or followed.

CAUTION

An operating procedure, practice, or condition that may result in damage to equipment if not carefully observed or followed.

Note

An operating procedure, practice, or condition that requires emphasis.

WORDING

Word usage and intended meaning throughout this publication is as follows:

"Shall" indicates the application of a procedure is mandatory.

"Should" indicates the application of a procedure is recommended.

"May" and "need not" indicate the application of a procedure is optional.

"Will" indicates future time. It never indicates any degree of requirement for application of a procedure.

FM ORIGINATOR

TO *(Primary Review Authority)*//JJJ//

INFO COMNAVWARDEVCOM NEWPORT RI//N5//

COMUSFLTFORCOM NORFOLK VA//JJJ//

COMPACFLT PEARL HARBOR HI//JJJ//

(Additional Commands as Appropriate)//JJJ//

BT

CLASSIFICATION//N03510//

MSGID/GENADMIN/*(Organization ID)*//

SUBJ/URGENT CHANGE RECOMMENDATION FOR *(Publication Short Title)*//

REF/A/DOC/NTTP 1-01//

POC/*(Command Representative)*//

RMKS/ 1. IAW REF A URGENT CHANGE IS RECOMMENDED FOR *(Publication Short Title)*

2. PAGE _____ ART/PARA NO _____ LINE NO _____ FIG NO _____

3. PROPOSED NEW TEXT *(Include classification)*

4. JUSTIFICATION.

BT

Message provided for subject matter; ensure that actual message conforms to MTF requirements.

Urgent Change Recommendation Format

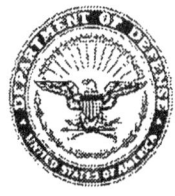

DEPARTMENT OF THE NAVY
NAME OF ACTIVITY
STREET ADDRESS
CITY, STATE XXXXX-XXXX

5219
Code/Serial
Date

FROM: *(Name, Grade or Title, Activity, Location)*
TO: *(Primary Review Authority)*

SUBJECT: ROUTINE CHANGE RECOMMENDATION TO *(Publication Short Title, Revision/Edition, Change Number, Publication Long Title)*

ENCL: *(List Attached Tables, Figures, etc.)*

1. The following changes are recommended for NTTP X-XX, Rev. X, Change X:

   a.   CHANGE: (Page 1-1, Paragraph 1.1.1, Line 1)
Replace "...the ~~National Command Authority~~ President and Secretary of Defense ~~establishes~~ procedures for the..."
REASON: SECNAVINST ####, dated ####, instructing the term "National Command Authority" be replaced with "President and Secretary of Defense."

   b.   ADD: (Page 2-1, Paragraph 2.2, Line 4)
Add sentence at end of paragraph "See Figure 2-1."
REASON: Sentence will refer reader to enclosed illustration.
Add Figure 2-1 (see enclosure) where appropriate.
REASON: Enclosed figure helps clarify text in Paragraph 2.2.

   c.   DELETE: (Page 4-2, Paragraph 4.2.2, Line 3)
Remove "Navy Tactical Support Activity."
"...the Naval War College, ~~Navy Tactical Support Activity,~~ and the Navy Warfare Development Command are responsible for..."
REASON: Activity has been deactivated.

2. Point of contact for this action is *(Name, Grade or Title, Telephone, E-mail Address).*

(SIGNATURE)
NAME

Copy to:
COMUSFLTFORCOM
COMPACFLT
COMNAVWARDEVCOM

Routine Change Recommendation Letter Format

CHAPTER 1

Introduction

1.1 MISSION

The mission of patient movement for health service support (HSS) is to minimize the effect that wounds, injuries, and disease have on unit effectiveness, readiness, and morale. This requires the HSS system to minimize morbidity and mortality for patients who cannot be returned to duty in a timely manner to an appropriate capability in or out of theater. Consistent with military and logistical operations, HSS operates in a continuum across strategic, operational, and tactical levels and pertains to deployed forces and their sustaining bases. Commanding officers (COs) effectively use their resources to treat, evacuate, and return to duty sick, injured, and wounded Marines and Sailors.

1.2 PATIENT MOVEMENT

The patient movement system provides a continuum of care, and it coordinates the movement of patients from the site of injury or illness using successive capabilities of medical care to a medical treatment facility (MTF) that can meet the needs of the patient. Patient movement consists of three components: medical regulating, patient evacuation, and en route care. The guiding principle is that patients are moved only as far rearward as the tactical situation dictates and as clinical needs warrant. Prompt movement of patients to the required level of clinical care is essential to prevent morbidity and mortality.

1.2.1 Patient Movement Across the Range of Military Operations

The execution of military missions in today's environment entails a joint force structure. The overarching planning process and the consideration for HSS personnel in joint medical operations are discussed in Navy Warfare Publication (NWP) 4-02, *Naval Expeditionary Health Service Support Afloat and Ashore,* and Joint Publication (JP) 4-02, *Health Service Support.*

For a more detailed discussion of the planning process for operational forces, see NWP 5-01, Navy Planning, *and JP 5-0,* Joint Operation Planning.

Success in joint operations is driven by a mutual understanding of the joint force medical capability throughout the range of military operations (ROMO), which varies in size, purpose, and combat intensity and extends from military engagement, security cooperation, and deterrence to crisis response, contingency operations, major operations, and campaigns. Since today's US military security environment is often engaged in operations below the threshold of armed conflict, it must be capable of sustaining operations before and after major operations.

Across the ROMO, patient movement requirements vary according to the type and scale of operation. Initially, each Service is responsible for organizing, training, and equipping its forces to meet patient movement requirements. Evacuation can require any combination of air, ground, and sea resources. Establishing a seamless evacuation system requires close coordination among the Services on evacuation doctrine employment, concept of operations, modernization and sustainment of equipment and platform capabilities, and interoperability of patient movement items (PMIs).

For a more detailed discussion of the range of military operations, see NWP 4-02, Naval Expeditionary Health Service Support Afloat and Ashore, *and JP 3-0,* Joint Operations.

1.2.2 Patient Movement Tasks

Patient movement operations, like Service operations, are based on a common-language master menu of tasks, conditions, and measurement subsets for COs of the US Navy (USN), US Marine Corps (USMC), and US Coast Guard (USCG) to develop Service-specific mission-essential task lists. The Chairman of the Joint Chiefs of Staff Manual (CJCSM) 3500.04 (series), *Universal Joint Task List (UJTL),* and the Chief of Naval Operations Instruction (OPNAVINST) 3500.38 (series), *Universal Naval Task List (UNTL),* include patient movement tasks identified by the CO at the strategic, operational, and tactical levels.

CJCSM 3500.03 (series), *Joint Training Manual for the Armed Forces of the United States,* describes how mission-essential task lists are developed. Patient movement conditions and planning considerations are discussed in Paragraph 3.3. Specific patient movement tasks are listed in Appendix A.

1.2.3 Joint Support to the Combatant Commander

Intratheater operations are the movement of patients between points within a combatant commander's (CCDR) area of responsibility (AOR). Intertheater operations are the movement of patients from the CCDR's AOR to points outside a CCDR's AOR.

1.2.3.1 Intratheater Operations

The joint force commander is responsible for developing intratheater patient movement policies in coordination with Service component evacuation representatives. Serving regions in a single geographic CCDR's requirements, intratheater operations are conducted using forces assigned, attached, and made available for tasking to the CCDR. Patients enter the system at the point of injury or illness and are moved to capabilities of care within the theater. Patients are most likely to enter the joint system for evacuation and medical regulation at the theater hospitalization capability. However, casualties can enter at the forward resuscitative care (FRC) capability, depending on the type of operation and forces supported. Intratheater patient movement can require a coordinated effort among the Services, coalition MTFs and/or host nation (HN) MTFs, the responsible patient movement requirements center (PMRC), and Service component organic and theater evacuation assets.

1.2.3.2 Intertheater Operations

The United States Transportation Command (USTRANSCOM) directs policies and procedures for intertheater patient movement and identifies transport resources. Intertheater operations are global and serve the transportation needs of the CCDR outside the AOR and support the conduct of operations within the AOR. Intertheater patient movement is primarily conducted using airlift assets as long evacuation distances may preclude other modes of patient movement in supporting rapid evacuation out of the combatant command (command authority) (COCOM) AOR. However, circumstances permitting, other modes and airlift assets may be used for intertheater patient movement. Patients usually enter the intertheater system from a theater hospitalization capability for movement to a definitive care capability outside the theater of operations and eventually to the continental United States (CONUS). Intertheater patient movement requires a coordinated effort among the Services or HN MTFs, responsible PMRCs, global patient movement requirements centers (GPMRCs), and transportation agencies.

1.2.3.3 Civil Support

Within the National Response Plan (NRP), the *Emergency Support Function (ESF) #8, Public Health and Medical Services Annex,* provides the mechanism for coordinated federal assistance to supplement state, local, and tribal resources in response to public health and medical care needs. The Department of Homeland Security (DHS)/Federal Emergency Management Agency (FEMA) coordinate the implementation of *ESF #8* through the Assistant Secretary of Public Health Emergency Preparedness (ASPHEP). In a major public health or medical emergency, local transportation assets may not be sufficient to meet demand. State or tribal requests for federal medical transportation assistance are executed by *ESF #8* in coordination with *ESF #1, Transportation Annex.*

The National Disaster Medical System (NDMS) has three missions: emergency medical care, transportation of patients, and definitive medical care. Four federal partners support these missions: the DHS (the lead federal agency), the Department of Health and Human Services (DHHS), the Department of Veterans Affairs (DVA), and DOD (a supporting federal agency). At the request of DHHS, DOD coordinates and provides support for the evacuation of seriously ill or injured patients to locations where hospital care or outpatient services are available.

In conjunction with the NDMS Medical Interagency Coordination Group (MIACG), DOD is responsible for regulating and tracking patients transported on DOD assets to appropriate treatment facilities such as nonfederal hospitals. DOD coordinates patient evacuation from a collection point in or near the incident site to NDMS patient reception areas through the NDMS MIACG. The United States Northern Command (USNORTHCOM) facilitates and identifies requirements for joint patient movement and transportation issues through the MIACG.

For further information on federal assistance in response to major disaster or emergency, refer to tactical memorandum (TACMEMO) NWDC TM 3-07.7-06, Domestic Disaster Relief Operations Planning.

1.2.4 Patient Movement Definitions

1.2.4.1 Medical Regulating

Medical regulating is the action and coordination necessary to arrange for the movement of patients through the capabilities of care. This process matches patients to an MTF with the necessary HSS capabilities and available bed space.

1.2.4.2 Patient Movement

Patient movement is the act or process of moving a sick, injured, wounded, or other person to obtain medical and/or dental care or treatment. Functions of patient movement include medical regulating, patient evacuation, and en route care.

1.2.4.3 Patient Evacuation

Patient evacuation is the removal of a patient by a variety of transport means (air, ground, rail, or sea) from a theater of military operation and between HSS capabilities to prevent further illness or injury and to provide additional care and disposition of patients from the military health care system.

1.2.4.4 Casualty Evacuation

Casualty evacuation (CASEVAC) is the unregulated movement of casualties that includes movement both to and between MTFs.

1.2.4.5 Medical Evacuation

Medical evacuation (MEDEVAC) refers to US Army (USA), Navy, Marine Corps, and Coast Guard patient movement using designated tactical or logistic aircraft, boats, ships, and other watercraft temporarily equipped and staffed with medical attendants for en route care.

1.2.4.6 Aeromedical Evacuation

Aeromedical evacuation (AE) is the movement of patients under medical supervision to and between MTFs by air transportation.

1.2.4.7 En Route Care

En route care is the continuation of care during evacuation between HSS capabilities in the continuum of care with no clinically attributed compromise of the patient's condition.

1.3 TAXONOMY OF CARE CAPABILITIES

HSS is provided to expeditionary forces using an ascending taxonomy of care capabilities that provide a continuum of essential care starting at the point of illness, injury, or wounding and continuing through evacuation and en route care within the HSS system. Patient movement components are encompassed in the taxonomy of care capabilities. Patients are directed to a facility with the capabilities required to begin decisive intervention to preserve life, limb, and eyesight, such as patient regulating and en route care. Once stabilized, the patients are either returned to duty or transferred to facilities outside the theater of operations for definitive treatment. The concept of care capabilities involves a scope of services and capacity provided within the HSS system bound by the following four interacting factors:

1. Urgency of the patient's needs

2. Requirements for mobility of medical personnel and facilities

3. Capabilities, equipment, and supplies of HSS personnel

4: The workload at each capability level relative to its treatment capacity.

Figure 1-1 summarizes the taxonomy of care capabilities based on JP 4-02, *Health Service Support.* The North Atlantic Treaty Organization (NATO) retains the levels of care schema, which corresponds to the US taxonomy Levels 1 through 4 as stated in the Allied Joint Publication (AJP) 4-10, *Allied Joint Medical Support Doctrine.* In coalition or multinational operations, personnel from non-NATO countries could have different interpretations of levels of care. In such circumstances, evacuation of casualties through progressive levels of care may not occur and patients may arrive at an expeditionary medical facility (EMF) without receiving first responder or forward resuscitative care.

CAPABILITY	HEALTH CARE	EXAMPLE*
First Responder	Medical care rendered at the point of initial injury or illness	Self Aid/Buddy Aid Hospital Corpsman Marine Corps Lifesavers
Forward Resuscitative Care	Forward advanced emergency medical treatment performed close to the point of injury/illness	Ship's Medical Department Battalion/Wing Aid Station Shock Trauma Platoon Forward Resuscitative Surgery System Expeditionary Medical Facility Surgical Company Casualty Receiving and Treatment Ship Aircraft Carrier
Theater Hospitalization	Modular theater hospitals with medical and surgical capabilities required to support the theater	Hospital Ship Expeditionary Medical Facility
Definitive Care	Full range of acute, convalescent, restorative, and rehabilitative care	OCONUS Medical Treatment Facility CONUS Medical Treatment Facility Veterans Administration National Disaster Medical Systems Hospital
En Route Care	Medical treatment during movement between capabilities	Tactical En Route Care Teams**
* This is not an all-inclusive list of medical resources. ** En route care can be used throughout all capabilities of care.		

Figure 1-1. Taxonomy of Care Capabilities

CHAPTER 2

Patient Movement Operations

2.1 GENERAL

The patient movement system provides access to the continuum of care and coordinates the movement of patients from the site of injury or illness through successive capabilities of care. To ensure the continuum of care and access the appropriate capability, Navy Medicine moves patients from shore to ship, from ship to ship, and from ship to shore. Patient movement consists of three focus areas or components: patient evacuation, en route care, and medical regulating. Prompt movement of patients to the required level of clinical care is essential to limit casualty, morbidity, and mortality.

2.2 CASUALTY EVACUATION

CASEVAC includes the tasks associated with the movement and ongoing treatment of the sick, wounded, and injured from the point of injury or illness to an MTF. In the absence of medical transport, any method of transportation may be used to evacuate casualties. The casualty may have received care ranging from buddy aid to forward resuscitative care and management during transportation.

2.3 NAVY FORCES

2.3.1 Navy Expeditionary Forces Ashore

Navy forces (NAVFOR) ashore use organic capabilities to accomplish casualty and medical evacuation. If the capability is unavailable, then the inherent Army or Marine Corps HSS structure is utilized. Refer to Chapter 4 for information on Navy patient movement operations and Appendix B for HSS capabilities.

2.3.2 Navy Forces Afloat

When a patient's health care needs exceed the capabilities of the ship providing primary support, patients are regulated to a higher capability of care as determined by the senior medical department representative (SMDR). Patient movement afloat consists of the full spectrum of patient movement, including medical regulating and patient evacuation. Generally patient movement afloat is located within two HSS structures: strike group operations and dispersed or independent operations. (See Figure 2-1 for a depiction of Navy patient movement flow in theater.)

2.3.2.1 Strike Group Operations

The inherent FRC capability within the expeditionary strike group (ESG) and carrier strike group (CSG) provides advanced medical care to the strike group. Patient movement is regulated through the afloat medical regulating system and is conducted through lifts of opportunity ranging from small boats to aircraft. If further patient evacuation is required, the ESG or CSG coordinates patient movement to the next capability of care. Predeployment planning is essential for determining available medical facilities and evacuation assets in the AOR. Prior to deployment, smart packs are developed for available medical facilities and evacuation assets.

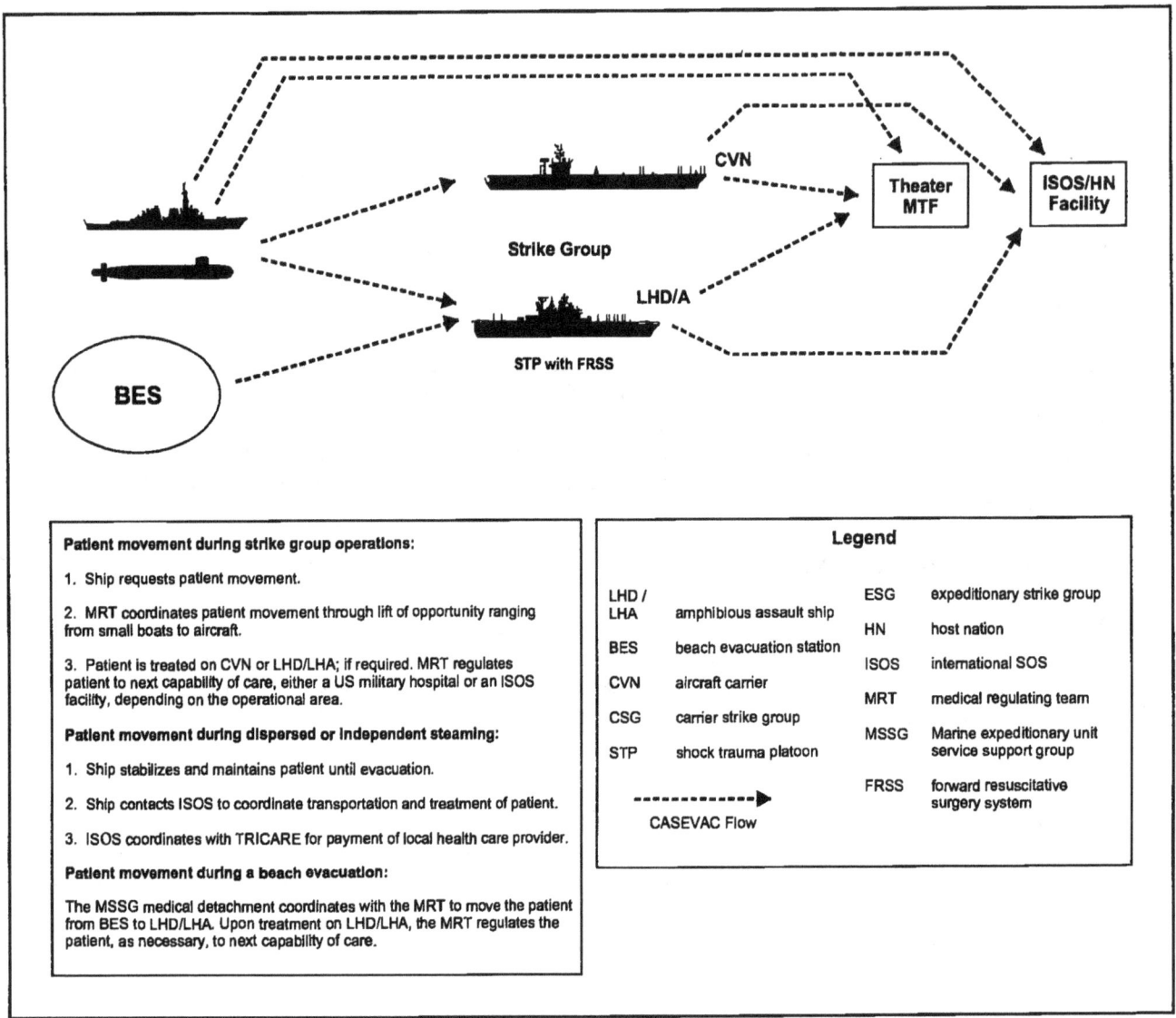

Figure 2-1. Navy Patient Movement Flow

2.3.2.2 Dispersed and Independent Operations

Patient movement for dispersed and independent operations requires extensive fleet planning and review of the operation order (OPORD) and evacuation policy. The ship's medical personnel stabilize and hold the patient until evacuation is arranged. Patient evacuation is usually coordinated with the contract provider TRICARE Global Remote Overseas (TGRO) or with a theater military MTF. (See Paragraph 2.5 for additional information about health care in remote locations.)

2.4 MARINE CORPS FORCES

The Marine Corps organization for combat is based on its unique force structure. HSS is a mission area common to every Marine air-ground task force (MAGTF) regardless of the mission. Definitive operational planning for HSS is always an integral part of all MAGTF operations. The inherent flexibility of the MAGTF and the broad spectrum of the potential MAGTF mission call for equal flexibility in HSS execution. The size, type, and configuration of HSS capabilities needed to effectively support a MAGTF is determined by mission, enemy, terrain and weather, troops and support available—time available (METT-T).

The theater commander may impose a patient skip policy, moving the patient past the next capability of care to a theater hospitalization capability. (See Figure 2-2 for a depiction of Marine Corps patient movement flow.) Chapter 5 provides specific information on Marine Corps patient movement operations. For further information on Service HSS capabilities, refer to Appendix B.

2.5 HEALTH CARE IN REMOTE LOCATIONS

Units operating in remote locations fall under the direction of the CCDR and the appropriate OPORD. In general, in a country or territory served by a DOD MTF, the MTF is contacted to determine its ability to care for the patient. At sea, when no US military health care MTF exists, it is customary to evacuate the ill and injured to non-US health care facilities in foreign countries. The TGRO provides urgent and emergent health care through health care contracts and is available to active duty service members regardless of their parent command and TRICARE enrollment status.

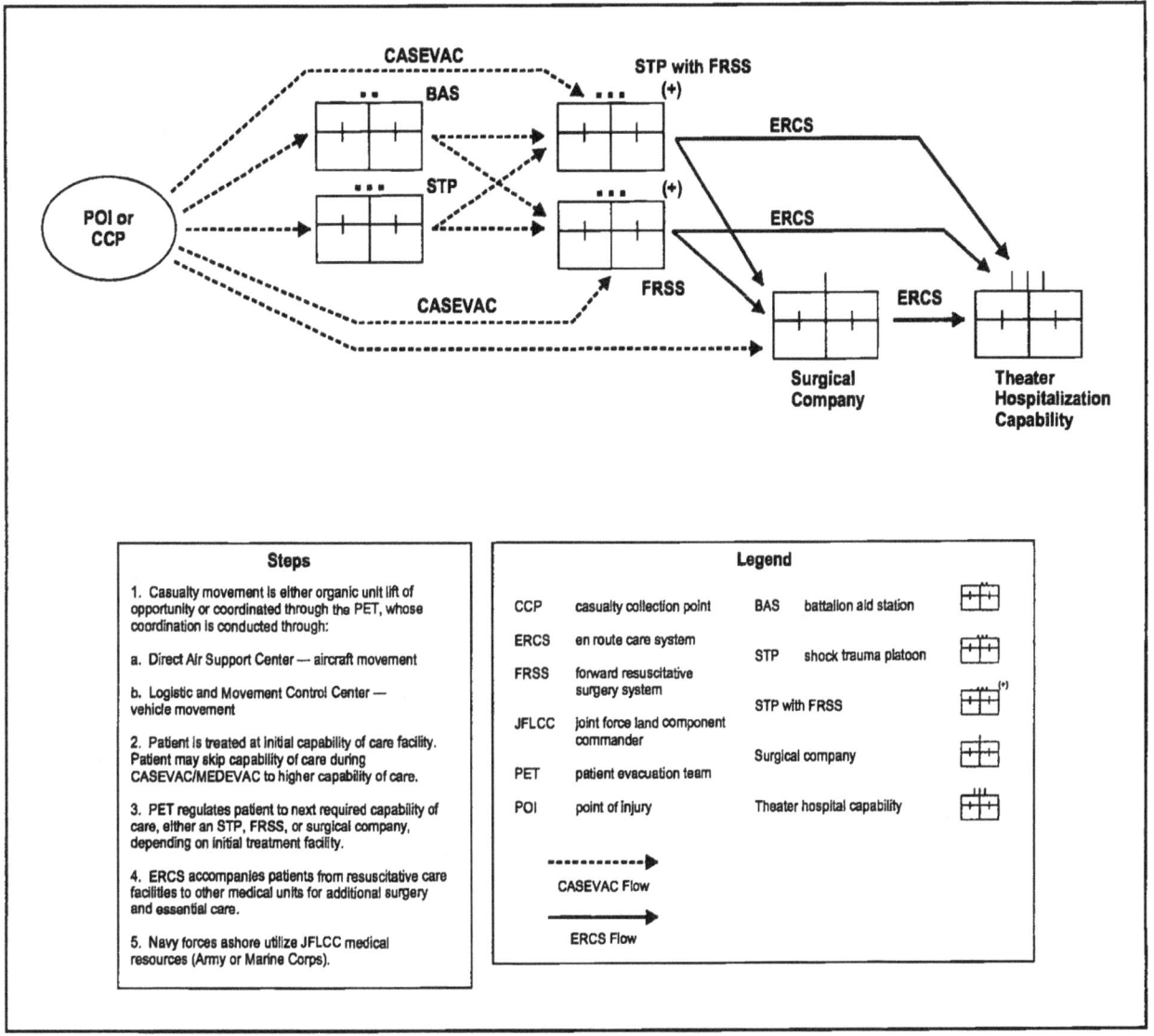

Figure 2-2. Marine Corps Patient Movement Flow

2.6 PATIENT MOVEMENT AND JOINT CAPABILITIES OF CARE

2.6.1 Point of Injury or Illness to Forward Resuscitative Care Capability Operations

The component commands are responsible for CASEVAC from point of injury or illness to casualty treatment stations, and for casualty movement from the first responder capability to FRC capabilities. CASEVAC is accomplished through dedicated, designated, or opportune ground or air transportation provided by a combination of litter carries, manual carries, ground transportation, and limited air transport (fixed- or rotary-wing). The Army employs dedicated patient evacuation assets such as ground and air ambulances. If Air Force assets are required at this level, lifts of opportunity may be used.

For more information on the use of Air Force assets, see JP 4-02, Health Service Support.

2.6.2 Forward Resuscitative Care Capability to Theater Hospitalization Capability

Movement from FRC capabilities is a Service component responsibility. Some operations may require evacuation by the joint common-user patient movement system. The Navy does not operate dedicated evacuation vehicles with the capacity to retrieve casualties from the FRC capability and evacuate to theater hospitalization. Requests for the joint common-user patient movement system are submitted to the joint patient movement requirements center (JPMRC) for coordination of casualty movement.

2.6.3 Theater Hospitalization Capability to Definitive Care Capability Operations

If a patient cannot be returned to duty within the limits of the theater patient movement policy, the originating MTF usually requests a patient to be moved to another MTF for more definitive care and disposition. The originating MTF will submit a patient movement request (PMR), in accordance with prescribed procedures using the USTRANSCOM medical regulating system or other prescribed communications systems. PMRs are submitted to an established JPMRC, which validates and regulates movement requirements and coordinates with the theater patient movement requirements center (TPMRC) for intratheater patient movement or with the GPMRC for intertheater patient movement.

The JPMRC identifies intratheater patient movement requirements through the joint movement control center (JMCC) to the air mobility division's aeromedical evacuation control team (AECT), and the TPMRC coordinates with the theater air mobility operations control center to identify theater airlift assets available. The TPMRC also coordinates with the GPMRC to identify intertheater patient movement requirements through the USTRANSCOM joint mobility control group.

2.6.4 First Responder/Forward Resuscitative Care Capability to Definitive Care Capability

Some joint operations present unique situations when a theater hospitalization capability does not exist. Stabilized casualties enter the joint common-user patient movement system near the first level of formalized medical care and are evacuated directly to a definitive care capability in another theater. In such cases, the component command medical regulating officer submits a PMR to the JPMRC. Movement within CONUS includes redistribution of patients to their home or unit of record. Members discharged from medical care who require movement to their home station instead of the theater are managed through the personnel system in a duty passenger status. The actual process varies and is documented in the OPORD.

CHAPTER 3

Patient Movement Planning

3.1 GENERAL

To be effective, the patient evacuation effort must be well planned and its execution synchronized. This chapter addresses patient evacuation under varying conditions and planning considerations where HSS personnel must be flexible and ready to improvise to meet the demands of unique conditions that present themselves in the operational environment.

3.2 PATIENT MOVEMENT EVACUATION CONSIDERATIONS

In the context of common joint military language, conditions are used to express variables of the environment affecting task performance. Conditions at all levels of operation are organized into three broad categories: physical environment, military environment, and civil environment. Patient movement may be the HSS capability most affected by conditions and warrants understanding and consideration in the operational environment. Planners must distinguish how environmental conditions affect the capability to perform patient movement by adapting the requirements to perform patient movement tasks (regulation, evacuation, and en route care) so that patient movement standards, such as those set by the commander, can be met. Paragraphs 3.2.1 thru 3.2.3 provide examples of conditions and subconditions used to define elements of the AOR affecting patient movement.

3.2.1 Physical Environment

The physical environment includes natural and manmade elements. The physical environment relevant to patient movement is organized in subcategories of land, sea, and air as follows:

1. Land includes terrain, geological features, manmade terrain features, and landlocked bodies of water.

2. Air includes tropical, subtropical, and arctic climates, and the seasons.

3. Sea includes ocean waters, the ocean bottom, and harbor capacity.

3.2.2 Military Environment

The military environment includes factors related to military forces, which include the following categories:

1. Mission

    a. Rules of engagement

    b. Commander's intent.

2. Forces

    a. Forces assigned

    b. Interoperability.

3. Command and control

    a. Joint/multinational

    b. Integration.

4. Intelligence

    a. Theater intelligence organization

    b. Medical threat.

5. Deployment, movement, and maneuver: Patient movement system responsiveness (theater evacuation capability)

6. Firepower

7. Protection

    a. Air superiority

    b. Land superiority

    c. Space superiority.

8. Sustainment

    a. Facility responsiveness

    b. Supply responsiveness

    c. Resupply responsiveness.

9. Threat

    a. Posture

    b. Opposing force size.

10. Conflict

    a. State of conflict

    b. Breadth of conflict

    c. Type of conflict.

3.2.3 Civil Environment

The civil environment includes factors related to populations, their governments, politics, cultures, and economies that impact military operations. The organization of civil conditions includes the following subcategories:

1. Political policies

    a. Domestic support

b. Political support

c. Public support.

2. Culture

a. HN stability

b. Foreign government involvement.

3. Economy

a. Population

b. Size of military

c. Gross domestic product.

4. International economic position: Self-sufficiency in economic areas

5. Industry

a. Growth rate

b. Electric production.

6. National potential

a. Transportation

b. Telecommunication infrastructure.

7. Science and technology

a. Research application

b. Technology production.

3.2.4 Impact of Conditions

Patient movement in operational theaters involves transporting patients to the appropriate capability of medical care in a timely manner. Conditions that military forces encounter must be counteracted to successfully complete the patient movement task. During casualty reception, collection, and movement with en route care, HSS units mimic civilian emergency medical response models in reacting to and mitigating these different conditions through planning.

Initially in operations, HSS units deploy with the medical estimate and an understanding of the medical threat and then establish support commensurate with mission type and scale under existing current considerations. For example, the environmental conditions dictate plausible evacuation routes and required modes of transport with a timeframe dictated by the commander.

3.3 PATIENT MOVEMENT PLANNING CONSIDERATIONS

The ability to successfully support combat operations requires a thorough mission analysis, a terrain analysis, trained medical personnel, and a thorough HSS estimate. HSS planning follows the same course as planning processes for any other element of operational support. HSS planning must be accomplished in conjunction with overall operational and logistic support planning. The HHS section of the operation plan (OPLAN) or OPORD must provide specific instructions for evacuation not otherwise addressed in the unit's standard operating procedures (SOPs).

For further information on HSS planning, refer to NWP 4-02, Naval Expeditionary Health Service Support Afloat and Ashore; *Commander Naval Surface Forces Instruction (COMNAVSURFORINST) 6000.1,* Shipboard Medical Procedures Manual; *Marine Corps Reference Publication (MCRP) 4-11.1E,* Health Service Support Field Reference Guide (draft); *Marine Corps Warfighting Publication (MCWP) 5-1,* Marine Corps Planning Process; *Marine Air-Ground Task Force Staff Training Program (MSTP) Pamphlet 5-0.3,* MAGTF Planner's Reference Manual; *and Field Manual (FM) 8-55,* Planning for Health Service Support.

3.3.1 General Patient Movement Planning Considerations

As METT-T factors affect the employment of all units, the HSS staff must consider the basic tenets of time, space, and logistics that influence the utilization of patient evacuation assets. These considerations include:

1. Patient's medical condition

2. Estimated number of casualties and types

3. Type of weapon systems employed by the enemy, for assessing injury

4. Hospital bed requirements, anticipated patient load, and areas of patient density

5. Availability, locations, and types of supporting MTFs

6. Availability of patient evacuation resources

7. Fire support plan to ensure patient evacuation assets are not dispatched onto routes and at the times affected by the fire support mission

8. Road network and dedicated patient evacuation routes (contaminated and clean)

9. Weather conditions

10. PMI

    a. Theater PMI exchange policy/PMI centers

    b. Return of allied nation and multinational force PMIs.

11. Blood requirements and availability

12. Medications that require temperature control

13. HN support and agreements; types of services available by HN assets

14. Evacuation of military working dogs

15. Special operations forces

    a. Evacuation coordinated with theater special operations command

b. Sensitivity of identifying information

c. Separate theater evacuation policy.

3.3.2 Mountain Operations

Mountain elevations vary from 1,000 feet to over 16,000 feet and have rapidly occurring weather and temperature changes. Operations in mountainous terrain require procedure modifications to counteract the environmental impact on personnel and equipment. Factors considered in a mountain environment include:

1. Rugged peaks, steep ridges, and deep valleys

2. Few navigable roads

3. Reduced range of communication

4. Unpredictable and severe changes in weather

5. High-altitude physiological impact

6. Endemic diseases and environmental injuries

7. Decreased partial pressure of oxygen affecting patient respiration

8. Availability of landing zones (LZs)

9. Altitude impact on rotary-wing lift capability

10. Survival and support techniques training.

3.3.3 Jungle Operations

Jungle operations degrade equipment and decrease personnel's ability to maneuver. Factors considered in a jungle environment include the following:

1. Few navigable roads

2. Limited availability of LZs

3. Extreme temperature and weather conditions

4. Endemic diseases and environmental injuries

5. Reduced range of communication

6. Decreased air pressure limiting rotary-wing lift capability

7. More frequent hoist operation requirements in thick jungle vegetation where LZs are unavailable.

3.3.4 Desert Operations

Deserts are arid and barren regions incapable of supporting human life. Temperatures range from above 136 degrees Fahrenheit (°F) to bitter cold. Day to night fluctuations in temperature can exceed 70 °F. Desert terrain can have mountains, rocky plateaus, and sandy dunes. Factors considered in a desert environment include the following:

1. Desert terrain and climate vary considerably from location to location. Medical intelligence should be obtained prior to deployment on operations conducted on desert terrain.

2. Units have long lines of communication and are widely dispersed.

3. Extra water is required for casualties to drink and to cool heat casualties.

4. Units must be able to treat environmental injuries unique to the desert.

5. The effects of wind and sand are interrelated. Sandstorms restrict visibility and hamper movement. Dust and sand present one of the greatest dangers to the proper functioning of medical and communications equipment.

6. Excessive heat adversely affects the following items:

   a. Vehicles and aircraft. Excessive heat causes vehicles to overheat, leading to greater than normal wear. Aircraft temperature limitations may be reached quickly, resulting in limited use during the hotter parts of the day.

   b. Medical supplies. Heat causes medical supplies to deteriorate. The shelf life of some medical supplies decreases when stored in hot climates.

   c. Medical equipment. Medical equipment must be protected from the effects of heat. It may be protected using the same techniques as those used to protect communications equipment.

3.3.5 Extreme Cold Weather Operations

Operations in the extreme cold have many of the limiting factors found in desert operations. The tundra and glacial areas are harsh, arid, and barren. Temperatures reaching lows of -80 °F to -100 °F combined with gale force winds make it impossible for humans to survive. Factors considered in a cold weather environment include the following:

1. Extended battle zones that increase evacuation distance and time

2. Extended maintenance for vehicles

3. Proper storage of medical supplies to prevent loss from freezing

4. Few terrain features or road networks

5. Extended hours of darkness at extreme latitudes

6. Unpredictable weather

7. Risk of environmental injuries

8. Regulating patient temperature while treating or awaiting transportation.

3.3.6 Patient Evacuation in a Chemical, Biological, Radiological, or Nuclear Environment

Evacuation of casualties in a chemical, biological, radiological, or nuclear (CBRN) environment forces the CO to consider to what extent medical personnel and evacuation resources will enter the contaminated area. The CO has flexibility in tailoring an evacuation system to meet the tactical situation and to deal with the CBRN environment. Factors considered in a CBRN environment include the following:

1. Mission-oriented protective posture gear, increased workloads, and the fatigue of battle greatly reduce the effectiveness of unit personnel.

2. Radiologically contaminated areas require operational exposure guidance.

3. Introducing uncontaminated aircraft into a contaminated area should be avoided. Ground ambulances should be used instead of air assets as long as their use does not adversely affect the casualty's medical condition.

4. Effects of weather and time upon contaminants should be weighed before action is taken.

3.3.7 Military Operations on Urbanized Terrain

Military operations on urbanized terrain (MOUT) are operations characterized by a three-dimensional battlefield with rubble, readymade fortified fighting positions, and an isolating effect on all combat and support units. The following factors are considered in an urban environment:

1. Using pulleys; special equipment used for lowering casualties from buildings or moving them from one building to another above the ground includes:

   a. Special harnesses

   b. Portable block and tackle equipment

   c. Lightweight collapsible ladders

   d. Grappling hooks

   e. Collapsible litters

   f. Heavy gloves

   g. Casualty blankets with shielding.

2. Reduced range of communication.

3. Alternate forms of communications, such as markers, panels, or field expedients (utility jackets or T-shirts) indicating the location of the wounded or injured.

4. Transportation operations within urban terrain are complicated and highly canalized by rubble and other battle damage. Strip maps of evacuation routes should be prepared, when applicable.

5. Medical personnel require special training in the TTP required to operate in a MOUT environment. They must be trained to cross open areas safely, avoid barricades and mines, enter and depart safely from buildings, and recognize situations where booby traps and ambushes are likely.

3.3.8 Infectious Patients

The Centers for Disease Control and Prevention (CDC) and USTRANSCOM are developing strategies for the movement of infectious patients. HSS units should contact the CCDR, the Service component, and USTRANSCOM for the latest guidance. Factors to consider when moving an infectious patient include the following:

1. Patients should be transported on a dedicated aircraft with the minimum number of crewmembers.

2. Infectious patients should be positioned as far downwind of cabin airflow as possible.

3. Mechanical ventilators for infectious patients should provide high-efficiency particulate air (HEPA) or equivalent filtration of airflow exhaust.

4. Whenever possible, noninfectious patients or passengers should not be on board.

5. The number of medical providers should be limited to those required to provide essential care during the flight.

6. Infection control measures should focus on source control; engineering controls to limit airborne dissemination of the virus; containment of the area of contamination, such as designating clean and dirty areas on the aircraft; use of personal protective equipment; safe work practices to prevent exposure; and waste disposal.

CHAPTER 4

Navy Patient Movement Operations

4.1 GENERAL

4.1.1 General Procedures

Patient movement procedures for Navy operations are established by the operational commander (numbered fleet) and promulgated through classified OPORDs to the ESG, CSG, and amphibious task force (ATF), three to six months prior to deployment. They remain in effect until superseded by new OPORDs or when the ship, ESG, CSG, or ATF is released or detached from the AOR. Upon entering the AOR, a set of OPORDs is promulgated by the numbered fleet responsible for that AOR. During wartime and peacetime, patient movement guidelines are dictated by the operational commander through the OPORD. All medical intelligence, disease occurrence, force health protection, patient care, and patient movement guidelines are found in the OPORD.

4.1.2 Intertheater Patient Movement Procedures

The Air Force has the lead role for intertheater patient movement. When the Air Force system is not a viable option, the TGRO treatment system can be used to MEDEVAC unless it is prohibited in the OPORD. TGRO designates a location for patient pickup; and the requesting unit transports the patient to the designated location, such as a beach, a port, or an airfield.

4.1.3 General Patient Preparation

Patients do not return to the unit once they leave the AOR unless there is a change to their medical condition and OPORD guidelines. Patients should take with them personal items of value, uniforms, and civilian clothes and should be advised that baggage restrictions apply (i.e., one bag and a small carry-on). Patients' personal protective equipment should be carried through patient movement; personal or issued weapons are prohibited. The unit can mail the remainder of the patients' belongings or hold belongings until the return to CONUS. General patient preparation is a function of the patient's chain of command.

The patient and patient escort should be briefed using the Afloat MEDEVAC Checklist. (See Figure F-1.) Information should include:

1. Where is the patient going? (Specific command.)

2. To whom does the patient report? (Specific person.)

3. What are the patient's restrictions? (Diet, ambulatory, 24-hour watch.)

4. Does the patient have records? (Ensure all medical/dental records, including labs and x rays, are given to the patient/escort.)

5. List points of contact (POCs). (MTFs, physician, Marine Corps/fleet liaison names and numbers.)

6. Who is the patient's emergency contact? (Immediate superior-in-command (ISIC), medical POC with number.)

7. Does the patient have a sufficient supply of medication? (Recommend a 7 to 10 day supply of medications for travel.)

8. Is all equipment in working order and properly labeled with medical department information? (Allows equipment to be tracked and returned to the ship as soon as possible.)

4.1.4 General Medical Department Preparation

Medical plans and tasks should be developed according to the OPORD issued by the CCDR. A copy should be obtained from the intelligence or operational officer and should include the following tasks performed by the Medical Department:

1. Develop message templates to report or request patient movement.

2. Develop medical smart packs (information POCs on medical facilities and patient movement assets) for each port and potential evacuation country or region.

3. Develop a complete MEDEVAC checklist if one is not provided in the OPORD, to include a list of personnel to notify in case of MEDEVAC. (See Appendix F for the Shipboard Treatment/Evacuation Team Checklist.)

4. Obtain early patient movement approval from the COC and from the patient's COC, unless a delay endangers the patient's life or limb.

5. Set up and practice MEDEVAC and patient movement scenarios.

6. Train the COC and crew.

7. Coordinate a MEDEVAC within the CSG/ESG/ATF through the strike group surgeon and accepting ship's senior medical officer (SMO).

8. Gain knowledge of key personnel who make the MEDEVAC process work.

9. Ensure that the following personnel-specific tasks are completed:

   a. The patient's COC provides uniforms, civilian clothes, personal items, passport, identification card, and escort.

   b. Personnel officers provide the patient's funded orders, unfunded orders, and travel arrangements in accordance with the OPORD guidelines and consider cash advancement from unit (disbursing).

   c. The air/operations officer sets up air or boat transfer.

   d. The communications officer notifies the accepting facility and external COC via message or e-mail through the SECRET Internet Protocol Router Network (SIPRNET).

   e. The weapons officer prepares elevators, if needed and available.

   f. The medical regulating control officer (MRCO) tracks the patient until final destination or return to unit.

10. Notify US Embassy defense attaché if the patient remains hospitalized in the HN.

11. Notify the husbanding agent of HN, and the medical representative will assist in arranging care, reports, and medical payment for services rendered.

12. Notify TGRO.

13. Notify the COC, medical COC, and next of kin (NOK).

14. Request the CO's final approval to MEDEVAC from ship.

4.1.5 Patient Movement Operational Risk Management

Personnel transporting patients should apply operational risk management principles in an environment of high quality situational awareness. Patients shall be stabilized prior to transport. The medical staff must ensure an adequate airway, stop bleeding, normalize blood pressure, immobilize orthopedic injuries, and plan for en route emergencies. For example, when an endotracheal tube displacement occurs, the attendant must ensure the use of proper equipment to reintubate. Knowing expected flight times helps to determine how much oxygen, intravenous (IV) fluid, and other supportive supplies are required.

Determine whether or not ambulatory patients should be made litter patients for comfort. To conserve batteries, oxygen, and other supplies, transport equipment should be reserved until prior to takeoff. A last check of the condition and vitals of each patient should also be executed and documented prior to transport. The patients being moved should carry all pertinent lab and x-ray records, including patient summaries. Physicians should communicate effectively, and other health providers should be familiar with aircraft types available. Patient movement personnel should consider environmental and operational challenges such as cold, hypoxia, vibration, noise, space limitation, diversion, and delay in planning.

4.2 PATIENT MOVEMENT OPERATIONAL PLATFORM SUPPORT

The medical regulating team (MRT) provides operational support for patient movement and is organic to the ESG. The ESG MRT coordinates seaward CASEVAC in the amphibious objective area (AOA) and patient evacuation within the ESG during periods underway. When control is sea based, units request CASEVAC via radio to the helicopter direction center (HDC) on the helicopter direction network. (See Appendix C for medical reports used by the MRT and Appendix D for status board formats used for patient movement.)

The MRT supports the following patient movement functions:

1. Developing a patient loading plan for casualty receiving and treatment ships (CRTSs)

2. Coordinating patient movement to HSS facilities

3. Establishing procedures for initiating radio or message traffic regarding patient evacuation

4. Receiving and transmitting information regarding HSS capabilities, patient evacuation status, and other information over the medical regulating network

5. Maintaining a spot status board on HSS facility status and capabilities

6. Developing the predeployment medical smart pack (hospitalization, blood supply, medical logistics, and health care personnel)

7. Monitoring and charting medical asset locations in theater, to include joint and coalition forces

8. Maintaining contact information for all theater medical assets.

4.2.1 Medical Regulating Team Structure

The MRT is part of the fleet surgical team (FST) staff within the ESG and maintains an informational relationship with the Marine expeditionary unit (MEU). It is located with the movement control agency (MCA) and can also be located with other units to facilitate patient movement.

4.2.2 Medical Regulating Team Staffing

The MRT staff consists of four medical personnel from the FST:

1. An MRCO who is a Navy Medical Service Corps (MSC) officer trained in medical regulating

2. Three medical regulating clerks, including one chief petty officer, who are enlisted corpsmen trained in medical regulating.

4.2.3 Roles and Responsibilities of Medical Regulating Team Personnel

1. Medical regulating control officer. Working closely with the MEU to coordinate the theater patient movement plan, the MRCO:

   a. Has overall responsibility for the MRT

   b. Coordinates the work of the MRT

   c. Establishes and maintains close liaisons among direct air support center (DASC) officers, the air operations officer, combat cargo, the administration department, MTF units, facilities in theater, and theater patient movement command and control (C2) elements.

2. Medical regulating clerk. The medical regulating clerk performs the following tasks:

   a. Monitors and communicates on the medical regulating network (MEDREGNET), the SIPRNET and Non-Secure Internet Protocol Router Network (NIPRNET) e-mails, the secure field telephone, and the iridium (satellite) phone

   b. Updates patient movement log and electronic facility spot status boards

   c. Updates theater HSS assets files for the MRT

   d. Prints and files hard copies of the patient movement log and electronic facility spot status board.

4.3 PATIENT MOVEMENT COMMUNICATION PLAN

The MEDREGNET secure chat provides rapid communications among the MRCO afloat, the patient evacuation officer (PEO) ashore, MRTs, patient evacuation clerks, and the joint/theater patient movement requirements center (J/TPMRC). It ensures that the MRCO and PEO have current information on the capabilities and status of HSS facilities supporting the operation. The MEDREGNET must be used for patient movement, medical supplies, blood reporting, and blood and blood product requests within the area of operations (AO). Units comprising the network are predesignated in the OPLAN/OPORD.

4.4 PATIENT MOVEMENT OPERATIONS

The ship's CO and SMO or its independent duty corpsman (IDC) must approve a patient's movement off the vessel. The SMO, or IDC, must balance the patient's condition with availability of en route care, urgency of treatment, and proposed aircraft altitude and flight time.

4.4.1 Independent Ships and Submarines

During patient movement to a shore medical facility, either the SMO or the IDC performs the following:

1. Determines whether or not the patient requires a MEDEVAC

2. When patients are moved to an MTF, the SMO or the IDC performs the following:

   a. Coordinates with the medical fleet liaison to establish direct communication between the ship's SMO and the accepting shore medical facility physician

   b. Sends the patient consult to the accepting physician

   c. Contacts fleet liaison

      (1) To verify readiness in order to receive the patient

      (2) To establish that the transportation of the patient from the rendezvous point to the hospital has occurred.

   d. Identifies a POC from the medical team standing by to receive the patient and the patient's accompanying medical documentation.

3. When patient movement is to an international medical facility, the SMO or the IDC performs the following:

   a. Follows guidelines for use by TGRO

   b. Determines when patients are litter or ambulatory and the requirements for medical attendants, medical equipment, and supplies.

4. Coordinates MEDEVAC with air operations and operations officer

5. Ensures that patients are delivered to the flight deck with required documentation

6. Composes and submits MEDEVAC message

7. Tracks patients' diagnoses, ships, referring physicians, current statuses, locations, and final dispositions.

4.4.2 Carrier Strike Group

The CSG uses the carrier-based SMO and the medical administrative officer (MAO). The carrier SMO is a CSG surgeon who coordinates patient movement with the MAO within the CSG. The ship's CO and SMO or its IDC determines the requirement for patient movement and initiates the request for movement to the carrier. Appendix E provides guidance on casualty categories and prioritization.

4.4.3 Strike Group Operations

4.4.3.1 Receiving Patients Afloat

1. Patients' ship. The transferring provider has notified the COC of the need to MEDEVAC. The ship's combat information center (CIC) or its officer of the deck notifies the ESG or CSG tactical action officer (TAO) and combat information center watch officer (CICWO) using chat or secured radio communication. The TAO and CICWO notify the ESG or CSG surgeon, who then proceeds to the CIC.

2. Receiving ship. The receiving ship ensures the following:

   a. The ESG and CSG surgeons communicate directly with the transferring provider and agree to accept up to 30 patients.

   b. The transferring provider and ESG and CSG surgeons agree on the details of transfer regarding using litter or ambulatory, and requirements for medical attendants and medical equipment and supplies.

   c. The ship's SMO or IDC ensures the following:

      (1) Treatment facilities are prepared in accordance with assessed condition.

      (2) A triage medical team is assembled, if necessary.

      (3) The ship's CO and executive officer (XO) are briefed about the MEDEVAC.

   d. The patient is either brought into flight deck triage, well deck, or directly into medical as determined by the SMO in coordination with ESG combat cargo, air operations, and flight deck control. From the flight deck triage, the patient goes to main medical using the elevator when moving a litter patient and using ladder wells and passageways when moving an ambulatory patient.

   e. The MRCO or MAO performs the following:

      (1) Coordinates with the TAO, operations officer, and air operations officer to plan MEDEVAC, taking into account the operational situation and urgency of the MEDEVAC

      (2) Informs the ESG combat cargo and air department if a neck or back injury is involved to ensure additional precautions are taken when offloading the patient from the helicopter

      (3) Considers providing experienced stretcher bearers from the medical department

      (4) Receives medical record or patient consult form from transferring ship

      (5) Ensures patient belongings are received from delivery aircraft

      (6) Stays in close contact with air operations regarding arrival of MEDEVAC

      (7) Contacts a division when a flight deck elevator is needed for patient transport

      (8) Opens ramp door if patient transport will be made via the flight deck ramp

      (9) Returns stretcher, hardware, and personnel to helicopter for return to the transferring ship.

   f. The operations officer performs the following:

      (1) Coordinates with air operations to contact the transferring ship regarding type of aircraft used for transport

      (2) Contacts air operations regarding type of aircraft, time of arrival, and other pertinent information

      (3) Contacts ESG combat cargo regarding flight deck assistance and stretcher bearers

      (4) Coordinates ship movement to arrive at recovery rendezvous.

   g. The air operations officer ensures that a ready deck is available for aircraft recovery.

4.4.3.2 Patient Movement Ashore

The ESG and CSG surgeons, the MAO and MRCO, and the operations officer have the following duties and responsibilities for patient movement ashore:

1. The ESG and CSG surgeons perform the following:

   a. The ship's CO makes the decision that a patient needs MEDEVAC based on the recommendation of the surgeon.

   b. If movement is to an MTF, the medical fleet liaison arranges direct communication between the ship's SMO and physician at the accepting shore medical facility and sends the patient consult to this physician.

   c. If movement is to an international medical facility, follow guidelines for use by TGRO. (See Paragraph 2.5 for additional information about health care in remote locations.)

   d. Coordinate with primary providers to make the following medical determinations:

      (1) Litter v. ambulatory

      (2) Requirements for medical attendants

      (3) Requirements for medical equipment/supplies.

2. The MRCO or MAO performs the following:

   a. Creates and/or maintains the applicable AOR medical smart pack.

   b. Contacts the medical fleet liaison for MEDEVAC needs.

   c. Coordinates MEDEVAC with air operations and operations officer.

   d. Contacts fleet liaison to verify when the hospital is ready to receive the patient and when transportation from rendezvous point to hospital has been established.

   e. Identifies a POC from the medical team standing by to take the patient and ensures that patient records accompany the patient.

   f. Ensures patient is delivered to flight deck with required documentation.

   g. Contacts ESG combat cargo or air operations who will be loading the patient onto the helicopter.

   h. Tracks patient, diagnosis, ship, referring physician, current status, location, and final disposition.

   i. Composes and submits the MEDEVAC message.

   j. If the patient is from the ship's company, the MAO notifies the patient's COC. If the patient is from embarked units, the MRCO notifies the patient's COC.

3. The operations officer performs the following:

   a. Obtains location coordinates

b. Contacts air operations to ready deck and fuel

c. Based on medical severity, composes and submits operations report NAVY BLUE message.

4.4.4 Amphibious Operations

During the phases of a conventional amphibious operation, patient movement functions and respective agency responsibilities include a preparation phase, a commander, amphibious task force (CATF) surgeon, and a landing force (LF) surgeon.

4.4.4.1 Preparation Phase

Personnel in charge of planning and conducting medical regulating functions must closely coordinate their actions. The ATF surgeon (CATF surgeon) or LF surgeon (MEU surgeon), and supporting HSS staff must realize that patient movement depends upon coordination with other staff directorates besides HSS. The OPLAN and OPORD, including applicable appendices, must address medical regulating, patient evacuation, and en route care. Patient movement can only be accomplished with the support of other elements of the task force (TF) and LF.

4.4.4.2 Amphibious Task Force Surgeon

The ATF and MEU surgeons are responsible for the formulation of the Services' patient movement system. Their responsibilities include the following:

1. Addressing the patient movement system in the OPLAN to provide policies and guidance for the operation, including the theater evacuation policy when it is not stated in a higher echelon OPLAN.

2. Ensuring that a CRTS is designated in the OPLAN and has the necessary HSS augmentation assets on board.

3. Ensuring that the OPLAN communications annex establishes a MEDREGNET and procedures for the conduct of patient movement among ships of the TF.

4. Ensuring that the HSS plan and the air plan address requirements for the MRT/MRCO to be collocated with the aviation control agency and provide liaison or augmentation to the J/TPMRC to ensure reliable communications during operations. The alternate medical regulating control agencies and subordinate medical regulators must have the same relationship with the subordinate aviation control agencies.

5. Ensuring that the OPLAN identifies patient movement assets aboard the primary control ship (PCS) and secondary control ship (SCS).

6. Reestablishing and maintaining network control of the MEDREGNET until operational control (OPCON) is passed ashore to the commander, landing force (CLF).

7. Identifying and requesting personnel augmentation to staff the medical regulating system, including the J/TPMRC.

8. Requesting that the Air Force aeromedical evacuation liaison team (AELT) and mobile aeromedical staging facility (MASF) facilitate evacuations out of the AOA.

9. Identifying the ATF MRCO and other ATF patient movement staff members.

10. Ensuring that all members of the ATF patient movement system have been trained and understand the procedures employed in the patient movement system before being assigned as a team member.

11. Monitoring patient movement throughout the operation.

4.4.4.3 Landing Force Surgeon

The LF surgeon coordinates and plans LF patient evacuation and medical regulating to ensure a seamless transition with the ATF patient movement system. The LF surgeon must be prepared to assume patient movement responsibilities when OPCON passes ashore to the CLF. The LF surgeon:

1. Ensures the medical appendix of the LF OPORD addresses the patient movement system in sufficient detail to ensure a seamless transfer of the patient movement system ashore, when appropriate

2. Ensures HSS assets (organic HSS units) are clearly identified and move ashore with appropriate serials

3. Ensures the communications plan includes activating and operating the MEDREGNET

4. Ensures the air plan and embarkation plan contain provisions for collocating the LF PEO and alternate LF PEO with the primary and alternate air control agencies, respectively

5. Ensures patient movement personnel are assigned to each HSS facility ashore and that they embark on the same ship/boat and land in the same serial as that unit

6. Ensures procedures are in place that permit the LF command post to alert the LF PEO of large numbers of patients being evacuated from the forward areas

7. Ensures the G/S-3 (operations) coordinates task organization and the landing plan, the G/S-4 (logistics) for embarkation, air officer for helicopter operations, and the G/S-6 (communications) officer for communication support

8. Ensures all members of the LF patient evacuation team (PET) have been trained and understand the proper procedures for patient movement.

9. Ensures that Monitors patient movement throughout the operation.

4.4.4.4 Ensures that Patient Movement Preparations

Initial preparations and placement of patient movement personnel takes place within the ATF and LF. Patient movement within the ATF includes the following preparations:

1. The MRCO and MRT are located on the CATF flagship and are collocated with the ATF surgeon. An alternate MRT located on the ship is designated as the alternate tanker airlift control center (TACC). Liaison or augmentation is provided to the JPMRC or TPMRC. The MRT has direct access to the MEDREGNET, functions as network control until control is transferred ashore, and is collocated with the aviation control agency of the TF.

2. The MRT is located on the PCS, the SCS, and each CRTS with its supporting movement control.

3. The PCS and SCS have an MRT located in or near the CIC. If the MRT is located outside the CIC, the MRT must have effective and reliable communications with the CIC. The MRT must receive current information regarding patients requiring surface craft evacuation to a CRTS or the use of service craft to evacuate patients. After receiving information from the MRCO, the MRT informs the PCS and SCS staff of the primary and secondary destinations for patients requiring evacuation.

4. The MRCO determines the need and location for other afloat MRTs and makes recommendations to the ATF surgeon. Any ship that can receive patients may have an MRT assigned. If the ship receiving patients is not equipped to properly care for them, the MRT notifies the MRCO, who arranges for the transfer of the patients to a CRTS.

5. The MRCO, in conjunction with the ATF surgeon, develops a patient loading plan for the ATF CRTS(s).

6. The MRCO develops procedures for transporting patients to HSS facilities.

7. The MRCO establishes procedures for initiating either radio or message traffic regarding patient evacuation.

8. The MRCO receives and transmits information regarding HSS capabilities, patient evacuation status, and other information over the MEDREGNET.

9. The MRCO maintains a spot status board on HSS facility status and capabilities.

10. The ship medical department notifies the MRCO whenever a change in status occurs in their department, such as a change in new patient or transferred patient status.

4.4.4.5 Patient Movement Preparation Within the Landing Force

1. The MAGTF logistics combat element (LCE) provides patient evacuation personnel assets (LF PEO and PET) for the LF.

2. The LF PEO embarks on the same ship and lands in the same serial as the LF DASC.

3. Once ashore, the LF PEO collocates with the LF DASC. If collocation is not possible, the location of the LF PEO is adjacent to that of the LF DASC. The LF PEO must have effective and reliable communication with the LF DASC.

4. The LF PEO guards the MEDREGNET and monitors requests for patient evacuation.

5. The LF PEO has reliable communication via the MEDREGNET with each LF PEO located at the various LF HSS facilities, with the LF alternate PEO, the ATF MRCO, and the J/TPMRC.

6. The LF PEO with the evacuation station communicates with the MRCO and may serve as a relay station when communications deteriorate between the LF PEO and MRCO.

7. The evacuation station has reliable communications with air and surface elements of the landing support battalion.

8. The alternate LF PEO's relationship with the alternate LF DASC is identical to the relationship between the LF PEO and LF DASC. The same requirements apply to embarkation, landing, location, and communications.

9. The LF PEO and PET monitor air and surface evacuation networks continuously and act on requests from network control for patient movement.

10. The evacuation station functions as the collection, triage, emergency treatment, and evacuation agent for patients received on the beach or in the LZ.

11. The evacuation station establishes communications with the beachmaster element helicopter support team.

    a. The LF PEO maintains a duplicate master facility spot status board for the LF.

    b. The LF PEO is prepared to assume the duties of MEDREGNET control when OPCON shifts ashore with the CLF.

c. The LF communications section provides the LF PEO and PET with the proper communication equipment, classified materials, publications, and supporting services.

d. The LF communications section provides the LF PEO with telephone connectivity to the LF telephone system.

e. The LF communications section provides communication links between the evacuation stations, beachmaster, and shore party commander.

4.4.4.6 Executing Patient Movement During Amphibious Operations

As ship-to-shore movement progresses, beach evacuation stations (BESs) and helicopter evacuation stations (HESs) are established at beach and landing zones and are collocated with the shore party and helicopter support team (HST) by the landing force support party (LFSP). The shore party or HST relays MEDEVAC requests from the BES or HES. Requests from the BES are processed by the PCS MRT via the MEDREGNET to advise the ATF MRCO of the requirement. The ATF MRCO recommends a CRTS that is capable of receiving and treating the casualties and the transportation mode. With PCS or helicopter support center (HSC) detachment concurrence for transportation, the PCS MRT advises the CRTS of incoming casualties and mode of transportation. Requests from the HES are processed by the primary HDC MRT via the MEDREGNET to advise the ATF MRCO of the requirement. The ATF MRCO recommends a CRTS.

A helicopter is normally provided for urgent and priority precedence casualties located at the HES. With HSC detachment or PCS concurrence for transportation, the primary HDC MRT advises the CRTS of incoming casualties and mode of transportation. Prior to the establishment of a BES or HES, casualties may be placed on-board helicopters or in medical boats as lifts of opportunity. In this case, the helicopter or medical boat advises the primary HDC or PCS of the MEDEVAC situation. The primary HDC or PCS acting on the advice of the ATF MRCO directs the helicopter or medical boat to a CRTS. CRTSs provide periodic facilities spot status reports to the ATF MRCO to maintain the master facility spot status board current. As the assault progresses, the LF establishes MTFs ashore to augment the CRTSs.

When hospital ships enter the AOA and are within helicopter range, the ATF or LF MRCO directs casualties to the hospital ship. When the LF medical regulating control center is established and air control has been passed to the DASC, control of medical regulating may be formally passed ashore to the CLF. With medical regulating control ashore, CRTSs and MTFs ashore advise the LF MRCO of their current capabilities through facilities spot status reports.

For further information on how Navy and Marine Corps planners execute the movement of personnel, equipment, and supplies from ships to shore in support of the landing force, see NTTP 3-02.1M/MCWP 3-31.5, Ship-to-Shore Movement.

4.4.4.7 MRCO Responsibilities During Amphibious Operations

The MRCO is responsible for the following tasks during amphibious operations:

1. Receive and validate patient movement requests through radio communication, secure e-mail or chat, Plain Old Telephone System (POTS), or fax.

2. Monitor patient movement activities and provide daily reports on matters such as patient movement issues, overall and daily patient movement, and information on specific patients (as requested).

3. Forward patient movement requirements to the appropriate transportation agency (LFSP and HDC) for patient movement mission execution.

4. Coordinate CRTS capabilities and patient status with the ship's MRT for patient movement for casualties and stabilized patients.

5. Establish or coordinate with the TPMRC for the appropriate destination treatment facility and mode of travel.

6. Maintain patient movement reporting and tracking procedures to include the following at a minimum:

   a. Reporting of available assets (lifts and beds)

   b. Designation of destination MTFs and an appropriate mode of transport

   c. In-transit visibility for both patients and related PMI.

7. Advise ATF surgeon on capabilities and limitations of supporting patient movement operations.

8. Coordinate with the ATF N-1 (Personnel) for mutual exchange of information.

4.4.4.8 Termination of Amphibious Operations

The CATF may withdraw with the concurrence of the CLF when the forward line of own troops extends inland and the logistical support base is well established. At this point, responsibility for HSS falls on the CLF and is exercised through the LF surgeon. An AELT attached to the MASF can be assigned to assist the LF. Patient evacuation and regulating out of theater will be coordinated with the TPMRC.

4.4.5 Navy Forces Ashore

NAVFOR ashore utilize the medical resources of the Army or Marine Corps JFLCC and have been combined under the Navy Expeditionary Combat Command (NECC), the functional command that centrally manages current and future readiness, resources, manning, training, and equipping of the Navy's expeditionary forces. HSS personnel and equipment are organic to each component of NAVFOR ashore with a range of medical capabilities including first responder and forward resuscitative care. The range of medical capabilities is accomplished by a hospital corpsman and medical officers assigned to the unit, and by the establishment of a battalion aid station (BAS) when deployed. The medical department organization consists of an SMO/SMDR, a hospital corpsman, and litter bearers.

CHAPTER 5

Marine Corps Patient Movement Operations

5.1 GENERAL

Patient movement involves a synchronized system of evacuating patients only as far rearward in the continuum of care as the patient's medical needs dictate using limited HSS assets, with each asset complementing the capabilities of the others. Appendix E provides guidance on casualty categories and prioritization.

5.2 PATIENT MOVEMENT ORGANIZATION AND RELATIONSHIPS

5.2.1 Patient Evacuation Team

The PET is divided between a PET-main and a PET-forward (FWD), each located and functionally integrated in the DASC-main and DASC-FWD, which are in turn collocated with the Marine division (MARDIV) main and FWD HQ. Within each DASC, the PET coordinates with the assault support watch officer in the execution of immediate assault support patient evacuation missions. The PET receives requests for patient movement through a 9-line request. Using the information in the patient evacuation requests, the PET determines the means of patient movement and destination HSS facilities.

After determining the best means for evacuation, the PET requests air movement from DASC or informs the requesting unit to coordinate ground movement with the logistics officer and assists as needed. The PET informs the receiving MTF of the incoming patient evacuation mission, tracks all patient movement through completion of the mission, assists the MARDIV personnel officer with patient tracking, and informs the MARDIV senior watch officer of all casualties resulting from enemy action.

5.2.1.1 Patient Evacuation Team Structure

The PET consists of the operations section within the medical battalion and reports to the medical support operations center (MSOC) prior to deployment. The MSOC will maintain an OPCON relationship with the PET. The PET is designed to be located with the DASC, but can be located within other units to facilitate patient movement.

1. A PET can be located with the logistics and movement control center (LMCC) for ground patient movement.

2. A PET can be located with the tactical air control center.

5.2.1.2 Patient Evacuation Team Staffing

The PET is made up of eight Navy personnel from the medical battalion and is augmented, when deployed, with two Marine radio operators from the communications company, Marine logistics group (MLG). The PEO is two officers from a Navy medical department, medical corps, nurse corps, or MSC, who are trained in medical regulating. The senior officer also functions as the PET officer in charge (OIC). If other PETs are deploying, additional personnel may be required. It is the responsibility of the MLG health service support element (HSSE) to coordinate augmentation requests for additional support.

5.2.1.3 Roles and Responsibilities of Patient Evacuation Team Personnel

1. PET officer in charge. This position has responsibility for the PET and works closely with the MSOC to coordinate the theater patient movement plan. The OIC coordinates the work of the PET chief, patient evacuation clerks, and Marine radio operators, and establishes and maintains close liaison with the DASC officers, the MARDIV air officers, the MARDIV G-1, the PEOs of HSS treatment units and facilities in theater, and theater patient movement C2 elements. The OIC functions as the shift PEO and is responsible for all patient movement while on duty during the shift.

2. PET chief. This position is responsible for the enlisted Sailors and Marines of the PET and assists the PET OIC in administrative requirements, including personnel, equipment, supply management, and patient evacuation record keeping. The PET chief functions as the shift PEO while on duty and coordinates with DASC and MARDIV senior enlisted leaders.

3. Patient evacuation clerks. Six enlisted corpsmen, including one chief petty officer, trained in medical regulating are the patient evacuation clerks, whose responsibilities include:

   a. Monitoring and communicating on the MEDREGNET, SIPRNET and NIPRNET e-mails, the secure field telephone, and iridium (satellite) phone

   b. Updating patient movement logs and electronic facility spot status boards as new information becomes available

   c. Updating the PET's display map of theater HSS assets

   d. Printing and filing hard copies of the patient movement log and electronic facility spot status board

   e. Sending periodic updated patient movement logs to the MSOC via SIPRNET e-mail

   f. Assisting the shift PEO in deciding the destination HSS asset and means of transportation for all casualties within the PET's geographic AOR.

4. Radio operator and maintenance Marines. The PET includes one Marine radio operator and one Marine radio maintenance technician. The Marines are responsible for establishing/maintaining, packing, and troubleshooting all PET communication equipment and establishing/maintaining communication on the MEDREGNET.

5. PET medical regulators. The PET functions as a liaison with the theater medical regulating officers to obtain information for commanders. All PET medical regulators (PEO/OIC, PET chief, and patient evacuation clerks) maintain broad situational awareness of the following:

   a. Current tactical situation, including disposition of friendly forces, offensive posture, and hostile threats, which is predictive of casualty load and estimated geographic locations where casualties can be expected

   b. Evacuation and emergency medical logistics missions planned and underway

   c. Availability of en route care and CASEVAC team

   d. Dedicated and designated air and ground evacuation assets available

   e. Weather conditions (flyable or not) at HSS facilities and airfields where air evacuation assets are stationed

   f. Last 24 hours of situation reports from medical commands located in the PET's AOR

g. Location and status of HSS treatment facilities in theater, including LZ information and status, and status of specialty equipment and specialists at those facilities

h. Points of contact

i. Shared responsibility during their shifts for deciding the destination HSS asset and means of transportation for all casualties within that PET's AOR.

5.2.1.4 Patient Evacuation Team Table of Equipment

The PET table of equipment (T/E) allows clear communication with all medical elements within the battlespace. The PET guards the MEDREGNET at all times. An MRC-138 radio high mobility multipurpose wheeled vehicle (HMMWV) with its antenna or a field expedient antenna and AN/GRA-39 remote provides the required communication distance and power necessary for the MEDREGNET. Additionally, the PET uses SIPRNET medical regulating chat, SIPRNET and NIPRNET e-mails, iridium (satellite) phones, and the secure field telephone. Rolling stock includes one MRC-138 radio HMMWV for personnel transport with one M-101A trailer for gear.

5.2.2 Ground Casualty Evacuation Organization

5.2.2.1 Ambulance Driver

Ambulance drivers and medical corpsmen are responsible for the ambulance at all times. The ambulance driver performs maintenance on the vehicle and is responsible for reporting major deficiencies to the section chief or supervisor. The ambulance driver and corpsman perform emergency medical interventions and provide emergency medical treatment in addition to driving. The ambulance driver performs the following tasks to provide maximum safety and welfare for the patients:

1. Ensures the patient is secured to the litter prior to loading

2. Ensures operational readiness and responsiveness accomplished by maintaining and using authorized equipment aboard the ambulance, including:

    a. Litters

    b. Blankets

    c. Splints

    d. Medical expendables

    e. Flashlights

    f. Auxiliary fuel

    g. Decontamination equipment.

3. Ensures the required information, tools, and equipment are obtained to navigate to the pickup location, including a map, tactical overlays, map coordinates, a compass, and position locator equipment, when available

4. Prepares the ambulance for patient loading and unloading

5. Assists litter bearers in patient loading and unloading

6. Performs property exchange when patients are loaded or unloaded

7. Provides emergency transport of medical personnel, medical supplies, and blood and blood products

8. Acts as a messenger for medical channels.

5.2.2.2 Hospital Corpsman as Assistant Driver

The hospital corpsman acts as an assistant driver and performs the following duties:

1. Reviews information on the field medical card (FMC) and becomes familiar with the condition of each patient being evacuated

2. Coordinates with individual(s) in charge for special instructions in the care and treatment of patients en route

3. Provides emergency medical treatment

4. Provides periodic checks of patients while en route

5. Supervises and assists in loading and unloading the ambulance

6. Assists the ambulance driver with land navigation and guides the driver when backing and moving off roads and when under blackout conditions.

5.2.3 Air Casualty Evacuation Organization

The air CASEVAC organization coordinates CASEVAC activities with other combat units, administrates supply requirements of the CASEVAC medical team, maintains CASEVAC mission records, and manages a quality assurance process for continuing improvement in CASEVAC operations.

5.2.3.1 CASEVAC Medical Team

The core of CASEVAC medical operations is the CASEVAC medical team, which consists of two or more providers staffing the CASEVAC aircraft. The CASEVAC medical team is responsible for the following:

1. Ensures CASEVAC aircraft is properly equipped to carry out the CASEVAC mission

    a. All gear on the minimal equipment list is loaded on the aircraft.

    b. All battery-powered equipment is fully charged.

    c. All oxygen tanks are full.

    d. Litters are appropriately configured for efficient loading and unloading of patients.

    e. All medical flight gear and medical equipment are fully functional.

2. Completes CASEVAC run sheets in a timely and accurate fashion

3. Triages and manages the patient load

4. Communicates relevant patient information to the pilot in command

5. Makes recommendations if deviation from the destination is issued by the DASC/PET

6. Assists in the patient loading and unloading

7. Assists in managing the LZ.

5.2.3.2 CASEVAC Team Leader

During each shift, one corpsman assumes the role of medical team leader. The medical team leader is directly responsible for supervising the conduct of all CASEVAC missions during the shift and for ensuring the missions proceed smoothly. The team leader assumes the following additional responsibilities:

1. Supervises the turnover of all CASEVAC gear during the change of shift, including maintaining all logs for narcotics and gear transfer

2. Ensures the prompt replenishment of supplies expended during CASEVAC missions

3. Ensures all battery-powered medical equipment is charging when not in use or staged aboard aircraft

4. Monitors aeromedical factors in all CASEVAC pilots and aircrew and reports signs of fatigue to the CASEVAC surgeon.

5.2.3.3 CASEVAC Leading Petty Officer

The leading petty officer (LPO) of the CASEVAC squadron's medical department normally holds the position of CASEVAC LPO and is appointed by the CASEVAC surgeon. When CASEVAC operations within a region involve only one squadron, the squadron's CASEVAC LPO may fill the responsibilities of the AOR CASEVAC LPO. The CASEVAC LPO's duties include the following:

1. Creates and submits schedules for medical teams to the squadron's operations department to be added to the squadron's daily flight schedule.

2. Collects and compiles all CASEVAC run sheets.

3. Collects and maintains statistics of all CASEVAC providers pertaining to flight time, number of missions flown, number of patients cared for, and instances of patient management that required a high level of medical skill, courage, and resourcefulness.

4. Ensures that the squadron's operations department maintains a current roster of all providers flying on CASEVAC missions. This roster must include the providers' names, ranks, and social security numbers so that all providers can be documented on a naval flight information record at the conclusion of each mission.

5. Supervises the squadron's stock of CASEVAC equipment and supplies, and submits timely requests for replenishments.

6. Maintains custody records for storage and use of narcotics.

5.2.3.4 Wing Surgeon

1. Roles and responsibilities of the wing surgeon include the following:

   a. Provides leadership and supervision to all medical providers participating in a squadron's CASEVAC mission.

   b. May fill the responsibilities of the AOR CASEVAC surgeon when CASEVAC operations within a region involve one squadron.

c. Ensures that all medical care rendered during CASEVAC missions meets the standards of care appropriate for the environment.

d. Collects and reviews CASEVAC run sheets.

e. Identifies problems encountered during missions and develops solutions to the problems.

f. Collects and disseminates MTF information to medical providers and the squadron operations department. MTF information includes locations and capabilities of forward resuscitative care, theater hospitalization facilities in the region, and the availability of a subspecialty at only one site. This information directly impacts in-flight triage and subsequent flight vectoring decisions.

g. Forwards CASEVAC run sheet data to the AOR CASEVAC surgeon or appropriate collecting agency.

h. Functions as liaison between the squadron and receiving medical facilities, especially when communications or patient transfer procedures fail.

i. Reviews selected CASEVAC missions with the PET with a goal of continually improving coordination and cooperation between the PET and CASEVAC team.

j. Reviews and supervises custody records for the storage and use of narcotics.

k. Ensures CASEVAC providers are prepared for missions by periodically assessing their level of medical knowledge, providing medical instruction on relevant topics, and debriefing complex missions.

2. Monitoring personnel professionalism. The wing surgeon should work to maintain an environment designed to constantly improve the CASEVAC system similar to the approaches of the Federal Aviation Administration (FAA) or Naval Safety Center. Encouraging the practice of self-reporting errors is a tool to prevent errors from being repeated. The wing surgeon should advise providers that reporting errors made in the conduct of a mission will not be met with disciplinary reprisal. Nonpunitive approaches to correcting errors or the events that led to an error will be pursued. While managing the providers on the teams, the wing surgeon may encounter individuals who do not possess the clinical capability, personality, or aeronautical adaptability to adequately staff CASEVAC missions.

3. Monitoring psychological stress. The wing surgeon monitors the psychological impact of missions on providers. The wing surgeon identifies a provider's psychological state, observes and identifies changes, determines underlying causes, and intervenes to reduce the level of stress the provider is encountering. In addition to operational fatigue, other stresses impacting the CASEVAC provider's emotional state include:

a. Guilt over a patient who died during transport

b. Nightmares triggered by the visions of profound trauma

c. Frustration that in-flight triage recommendations were not followed

d. Fear resulting from a flight that became dangerously close to hostile fire or mishap

e. Distraction generated by the provider's own uncertainty as to whether a particular case was managed appropriately.

5.2.3.5 Helicopter Aircraft Commander

The helicopter aircraft commander (HAC) is responsible for safe conduct and flight and mission success, and makes the final decision on where an aircraft travels. Medical personnel on board do not have final authority for where CASEVAC patients are delivered. To arrive at a destination decision, the HAC must consider aircraft factors, information provided by medical personnel, and information from the DASC/PET squadron intelligence and operations officers. Instances of medical teams failing to demonstrate respect for flight decisions made by the HAC or section leader should be reported to the appropriate level SMO or CO.

5.3 PATIENT MOVEMENT COMMAND AND CONTROL ORGANIZATION

5.3.1 Medical Support Operations Center

5.3.1.1 Medical Support Operations Center Responsibilities

The MSOC is staffed by the MLG HSSE and functions within the MLG command center (CC), which supports forward and rear CCs. The MSOC is responsible for the following:

1. Establishes patient evacuation procedures

2. Advises the commanding general and MLG

3. Facilitates the distribution of Class VIII (A/B) supplies

4. Collects, analyzes, and distributes medical data from all HSS units to higher authority and supported units.

5.3.1.2 Medical Support Operations Center Communications

The MSOC is the controlling authority for patient movement in the Marine expeditionary force (MEF). The MSOC has communication links with the following:

1. DASC

2. Subordinate elements

3. Surgical companies

4. Forward resuscitative surgery system (FRSS) units

5. Theater hospitalization MTFs

6. CRTS in the AOA.

5.3.1.3 Coordinating Patient Movement

1. The MSOC interfaces with the MAGTF air combat element (ACE) through the air liaison officer (ALO) in the MLG CC and the PET in the DASC. The MSOC or DASC provides aeromedical input into the planning and coordination of the patient evacuation mission.

2. For ground evacuation, the PET interfaces with the MSOC in the MLG CC and with HSSEs in the LCE HQ for efficient and effective patient movement.

5.3.2 Direct Air Support Center

The DASC is the principal air control agency for the direction of air operations directly supporting ground forces. It processes and coordinates requests for immediate air support, including medical evacuation, and coordinates air missions requiring integration with ground forces and other supporting arms. Additionally, the DASC serves as the primary processing point for all medical evacuation requests.

5.3.3 Marine Logistics Group Air Liaison Officer

The ALO is a naval aviator with a secondary function as an air officer/forward air controller. The ALO is responsible for providing aviation liaison to the MLG in all matters pertaining to intratheater airlift, air fires, aviation planning (including HSTs), and air delivery. The ALO supports the force protection/fires section for targeting, local security and close air support requirements, and the MSOC in patient movement; and registers air tasking order (ATO) requests for future designated patient evacuation standby aircraft.

5.3.4 Logistic and Movement Control Center

The LMCC is administratively located in the MLG CC and is the MEF's central agency for the coordination of ground transportation. The LMCC organizes, tracks, deconflicts, and manages all tactical passengers, cargo, and convoy movements within the MEF's AOR and coordinates patient ground movement.

5.3.5 Aeromedical Evacuation Liaison Team

The Air Force AELT provides support between the forward user and the aeromedical evacuation system (AES) in the form of operational and clinical interface. This support may occur at locations that do not otherwise have Air Force personnel, such as far forward/bare bases and shipboard. The flight nurse liaison assists the local medical unit to prepare patients for flight.

The administrative officer is responsible for working with the airlift center and aerial port elements to ensure that the aircraft is properly configured and that equipment pallets, patients, and support personnel are properly manifested on the AE mission. The communications personnel may be integrated into the airlift operations element supporting flight line operations or the wing operations center. Establishing a communication network with airlift operations is essential for rapid evacuation.

When an AELT is collocated with the MEF, the AELT is able to provide the following:

1. Communication link between MEF patient movement entities and the AES

2. Coordination of MEF patient movement requests and subsequent movement activity between the aeromedical evacuation control center (AECC) and the MEF

3. Reporting of requirements for special equipment and/or medical attendants to accompany casualties during flight.

5.3.6 Mobile Aeromedical Staging Facility

The MASF provides rapid-response patient staging, limited holding, and emergent AE crew support capability. The MASF provides forward support with the smallest footprint and is usually the AE element used in support of special operation forces. The MASF is located at or near airheads capable of supporting conventional mobility airlift and may be augmented with additional personnel and equipment to increase patient staging capability as needed. It can serve as the entry point of MEF patients into the Air Force AES when collocated.

5.4 PATIENT MOVEMENT COMMUNICATION PLAN

5.4.1 Movement

Primary communication for movement control and coordination is a combination of radio, SIPRNET (chat, e-mail, and web), and the secure field telephone. Point of wounding and BAS communication to the battalion command element is primarily through radio or field telephone. In addition, communication between the battalion/regimental COC and the DASC is through the tactical air request/helicopter request (TAR/HR) net or field telephone. The MSOC communicates with the DASC/PET, LCE HQ, and forward units through SIPRNET, secure field telephone, and/or radio. The MSOC maintains a command and control personal computer (C2PC) web-based map overlay that communicates current locations of all casualty care and movement assets.

5.4.2 Medical Regulating Network

The MEDREGNET is used as a communications link to pass pertinent patient information and to serve as a means of communication between all HSS units. The network is used for passing reports and spot status on FRC beds when other communication is not available. The PET, the LCE HQ, and the surgical companies should guard this network. The MLG MSOC serves as net control. Communications over the MEDREGNET are usually secure with frequencies published in the OPLAN or Annex K of the OPORD.

The MEF trains personnel assigned to perform patient evacuation/medical regulating functions, such as monitoring the MEDREGNET 24 hours per day, submitting reports, and maintaining medical logs. Patient evacuation personnel and the MEF must have reliable access to the MEDREGNET and establish internal procedures to monitor the network and to maintain required logs.

5.4.3 Patient Evacuation Team Record Keeping and Documentation

The PET maintains electronic and hard copy information documenting all activities, to include PET coordinated patient evacuation missions and information from the supporting HSS units pertinent to patient evacuation and medical regulating. Appendix C provides the medical reports utilized by the PET. The following information must be documented:

1. Watchstander information.

   a. Name

   b. Rank

   c. Duty times and dates.

2. Facility spot status board. A copy of a facility spot status board (Excel® spreadsheet) is saved electronically and printed at the beginning of each shift, every four hours, and periodically as facilities' statuses change significantly. Appendix D provides the patient movement status board formats.

The facility spot status board should be updated when the PET receives the following:

   a. A facility spot status report or medical situation report on any HSS asset

   b. Confirmation of a patient evacuation mission departing any HSS asset with patients on board

   c. Confirmation of CASEVAC or MEDEVAC mission arriving at any HSS asset with patients on board.

3. Mission tracking board. The following information should be recorded on a mission tracking board (Excel® spreadsheet) for all helicopter and ground evacuation missions:

   a. Date

   b. Time request received

   c. Time mission launched

   d. Ground/sea vehicle type

   e. Air dedicated/air lift of opportunity vehicle type

   f. Mission call sign

   g. Air request number

   h. Air mission number

   i. Number of urgent patients each mission

   j. Number of urgent surgical patients each mission

   k. Number of priority patients each mission

   l. Number of routine patients each mission

   m. Total patients each mission

   n. Pickup unit

   o. Pickup location grid coordinates

   p. Dropoff unit

   q. Pickup time

   r. Dropoff time

   s. Elapsed time from request receipt to dropoff

   t. Nationality of patients

   u. Miscellaneous remarks.

4. Reports. A copy of all reports obtained by the MSOC and PET must be saved electronically and the hard copies printed. The reports most relevant to patient movement are found in Appendix D.

5.5 PATIENT MOVEMENT OPERATIONS

5.5.1 Command and Control and Medical Regulating

This process refers to the movement of patients from FRC capability to theater hospitalization capability or higher facilities that have the necessary HSS capabilities and available bedspace. Medical personnel make patient regulating decisions.

5.5.1.1 Theater Medical Regulating

The theater commander may perform C2 from first responder capability through the definitive care capability by the theater MRCO, or as directed. The MLG health service support officer (HSSO) is responsible for coordinating with the theater MRCO for medical regulating patients from FRC capability Marine Corps MTFs to higher-level MTFs. Additionally, the MLG HSSO may be required to perform medical regulating until a J/TPMRC is established. Detailed information is listed in the OPLAN or OPORD (Appendix 1 to Annex Q and/or Appendix 9 to Annex D).

5.5.1.2 Seabased Medical Regulating

While C2 is sea based, the ESG MRCO is responsible for patient movement and medical regulating and coordination with the J/TPMRC.

5.5.1.3 Medical Regulating Ashore

When OPCON passes ashore, responsibility for evacuation of casualties is assumed by the accepting unit. The MLG HSSO is responsible for planning and coordinating casualty evacuation, providing trained personnel to function as the LF MRCO and PET to the control authorities for aviation and ground transportation, and providing medical regulation. The MEU medical planner/HSSO is responsible for coordinating the same with the ACE, the battalion landing team (BLT), and the combat logistics battalion (CLB).

5.5.2 Command and Control and Patient Movement

5.5.2.1 Theater Patient Movement

The J/TPMRC is responsible for coordinating intertheater patient movement (strategic AE and medical regulating) of casualties from theater hospitalization capability medical facilities. If an AELT is provided, it will be under the direction of the LF MRCO and utilized to coordinate fixed-wing intratheater and intertheater AE of patients. (See Appendix B for more information on patient movement transportation assets.)

5.5.2.2 Seabased Patient Movement

Requesting units make patient evacuation requests by radio to the HDC on the helicopter direction network when control is sea based.

5.5.2.3 Patient Movement Ashore

When command and/or net control has been passed ashore, requests will be directed to the DASC for MEF and Marine expeditionary brigade (MEB) operations and the air support element (ASE) or DASC for MEU operations on the TAR/HR network. The helicopter director consults with either the ESG MRCO when sea based or the LF MRCO, through the PET located in the ASE/DASC when ashore, for primary and alternate MTFs, location, availability, LZ coordinates, radio frequencies, and ensures the designated facility has the capability commensurate with the casualty's condition.

During MEF and MEB operations, the MLG HSSO, located in the MSOC of the combat service support operations center (CSSOC), supervises the LF MRCO, who oversees two PETs. The primary PET is collocated with the DASC; the secondary PET may be collocated with the LMCC, also in the CSSOC. During MEU operations, the LF MRCO is the MEU medical planner. The LF MRCO coordinates with the ESG MRCO, J/TPMRCO, and if provided, the AELT. The LF MRCO maintains the master medical facility spot status board, controls the MEDREGNET, and maintains the patient movement log. The LMCC PET is responsible for coordinating ground evacuations of casualties in coordination with the LMCC and supporting patient tracking. The LMCC PET maintains a duplicate medical facility spot status board and is prepared to assume the responsibilities of the primary PET.

5.5.3 Ground Casualty Evacuation

Based on the criticality of the casualties and the availability of air assets, the PET may direct casualty movement using ground assets. Rearward medical units go forward to pick up casualties. Ground evacuation is divided into two stages:

1. Stage 1 is movement from division units to the direct support (DS) LCE unit. The DS LCE unit has STPs, a FRSS, or combination of both. The PET will contact the LCE HQ in DS of division units and provide MEDEVAC request form information to coordinate ground transportation. The LCE plans and coordinates the movement with the regimental HQ and determines the requirements for an ambulance exchange point (AXP).

   Patients evacuated by ground transport to the LCE should be treated and either returned to duty or evacuated to the rear. The LCE HQ immediately notifies the PET and the MSOC of the disposition of the casualties over the SIPRNET, secure field telephone, or the MEDREGNET.

2. Stage 2 movement is from the DS LCE unit to the general support (GS) LCE unit with FRC capability. The PET contacts the MLG MSOC or GS LCE HQ and provides MEDEVAC request form information to coordinate ground transportation. The MLG MSOC/LMCC and GS LCE coordinates the movement with the DS LCE HQ and determines requirements and location for an AXP.

5.5.3.1 Ground Ambulances

Ground ambulances are vehicles designed for carrying patients, and are staffed with a driver/corpsman qualified in basic emergency medical treatment procedures. They are dedicated assets for the medical mission and are organic to HSS units that evacuate sick, injured, and wounded Marines and Sailors by ground ambulance.

The Geneva Conventions stipulate that ground ambulances be clearly marked with the distinctive Red Cross emblem on a white background. Camouflaging or not displaying the Red Cross emblem can result in the loss of the protections afforded under the Geneva Conventions. Guidance regarding the camouflage of medical units, vehicles, and aircraft on the ground is contained in Standard Agreement (STANAG) 2931, *Camouflage of the Red Cross and Red Crescent on Land in Tactical Operations.*

Field units may operate military field ambulances on paved and secondary roads, trails, and cross-country terrain. Field ambulances operating in the forward areas of the combat zone (CZ) must possess mobility and survivability comparable to the units being supported. Current field ambulance variations include the HMMWV D 1001 and the HMMWV D 1002 (soft 18 top). These ambulances are used to evacuate patients from frontline units to BASs.

5.5.3.2 Ambulance Loading and Unloading

In loading and unloading ambulances, litter patients are moved carefully. Details of the loading and unloading procedures vary slightly depending on the number of bearers, the presence or absence of a medical corpsman, and the type of vehicle. The procedures for ambulance loading and unloading are as follows:

1. Patients usually are loaded headfirst except when they have head injuries. Patients placed headfirst, in the direction of travel, are less likely to experience motion sickness, nausea, and noise from rear doors opening and closing. Loading patients headfirst protects them from further injury in the event of a rear-end collision.

2. When a patient requires en route care for an injury to one side of the body, it may be necessary to load the patient feetfirst to make the injured side readily accessible from the aisle. Patients with wounds of the chest or abdomen and those receiving IV fluids are loaded in lower berths to provide gravity flow. For ease of loading and patient comfort, patients wearing bulky splints should be placed on lower berths.

3. A three-man team is required to load and unload the ambulance. The sequence for loading four litter patients in the berths is upper right, lower right, upper left, and lower left.

4. The most seriously injured patients are loaded last to ensure they are the first to be taken out of the ambulance. The sequence for unloading is the reverse of loading.

5. The loading/unloading team must ensure that straps and equipment do not inhibit litter loading operations.

6. When patients are picked up from several locations, loading the least seriously injured patient first and the most seriously injured patient last cannot always be applied. A previously loaded patient should not be unloaded in order to maintain the loading sequence.

7. The receiving MTF must be made aware of the most seriously injured patients.

8. When loading more than two litter patients, the upper litter rack patients must be loaded first. Injury may result if litter patients are loaded in lower racks first.

9. When unloading more than two litter patients, lower litter rack patients must be unloaded first.

5.5.3.3 Rules for Employment of Ambulance and Ambulance Personnel

1. The use of ambulances is restricted to the transportation of the following three categories:

   a. Sick or injured personnel

   b. Medical personnel

   c. Class VIII supplies/equipment and blood.

2. Medical personnel assigned to the ambulances will:

   a. Adhere to the tactical CO's standards for uniforms, camouflage, and other requirements identified in the supported unit's tactical SOP.

   b. Participate in the medical training being conducted at the supported medical element.

   c. Assist with patient treatment.

   d. Perform preventive maintenance checks on vehicles.

   e. Ensure vehicles are restocked with required Class VIII supplies, full of fuel, and ready for the next evacuation mission.

3. Medical personnel assigned to the ambulances that are positioned with the supported medical element will not:

   a. Be required to perform duties such as mess duty, detainees or perimeter guards, or drivers of other than the assigned vehicle

   b. Violate the provisions of the Geneva Conventions.

5.5.4 Air Casualty Evacuation

5.5.4.1 Phase I

AE is the preferred method for transferring critically wounded patients whose survival depends on immediate surgery. Rotary-wing AE units initiate patient evacuation by submitting a standard NATO 9-line MEDEVAC request by radio directly to the DASC, the battalion, or regimental command element. These requests are then forwarded to the DASC over the TAR/HR network.

In conjunction with the DASC, the PET determines when aeromedical evacuation is used based on the patient's condition and air asset availability. The DASC records the information from the MEDEVAC request on an assault support request (ASR) form and then passes it to the PET. The PET reviews the spot status board and coordinates with the MSOC to recommend an evacuation mode and a destination MTF. The DASC personnel can accept or reject the PET's recommendation based on tactical circumstances and availability of transportation assets. If rejected, the PET coordinates with the MSOC or the LCE to recommend either alternative destination MTFs or the use of ground movement assets.

Coordination between the PET, DASC, LCE, and MSOC ensures that the patient receives appropriate care, that no MTF is overloaded, and that the tactical situation is not negatively impacted. DASC personnel record the destination MTF on their ASR form and dispatch a helicopter for the CASEVAC mission. DASC personnel will contact the battalion or LCE HQs and inform them of the estimated time of arrival of the helicopter at the designated LZ, relay any special coordinating instructions, and identify destination facility.

The PET notifies the MSOC and destination MTF over SIPRNET e-mail, secure field telephone, or MEDREGNET of the patient evacuation mission. Timely notification of the destination MTF is essential to ensure the PET can prepare to receive the incoming casualties and transport them from their LZ. The PET and MSOC will record required information in their respective patient movement logs and will monitor the casualty evacuation mission until the casualties are received at the destination MTF.

5.5.4.2 Phase II

The AELT will register the MLG requirements with the JPMRC, who will designate fixed-wing lift and a destination facility. Upon notification by the JPMRC, the AELT will notify the surgical company/MSOC/PET when the patient must be moved to the airfield or MASF for AE. The supporting LCE/MSOC/LMCC will coordinate the use of Marine Corps transportation assets (ground or air) to move patients to the designated MASF for evacuation out of theater.

Air evacuation is accomplished for urgent and urgent surgical category patients. Use of air assets for CASEVAC depends on METT-T. Within the MEF, the MLG HSSE, in conjunction with the MLG LMCC, plans for medical evacuation aircraft. In most cases, the limited number of aircraft in the Marine Corps inventory precludes the assignment of dedicated aircraft, which are externally marked with a red cross and reserved to support the MEDEVAC mission. All Marine Corps rotary-wing and utility aircraft have the capability to perform the CASEVAC mission. The effectiveness and efficiency of HSS is enhanced by air evacuation to:

1. Remove patients from otherwise inaccessible areas.

2. Circumvent fixed defenses and natural obstacles.

3. Deliver medical supplies and blood products.

4. Provide a means of rapid evacuation.

5. Provide emergency airlift of medical personnel, equipment, and supplies.

5.5.4.3 Landing Zone Considerations

LZs for CASEVAC operations are the responsibility of the supported unit. BASs are responsible for establishing the LZ for CASEVAC operations. LZ selection criteria for the CASEVAC LZ are location, marking, communications, capacity, and obstacles.

1. Location. The LZ must be in close proximity to the aid station but at a distance which will not interfere with aid station operations. Casualties may have to be carried by hand to the waiting aircraft. Establish the LZ downwind from the aid station, if possible, to prevent blowing dust on the aid station. A minimum distance of 150 meters should be acceptable to keep aircraft from interfering with aid station operations.

2. Marking. LZ markings must be visible from the air. During daylight operations the LZ can be marked using a visual signal (VS)-17 panel, smoke, or signal mirror. If a VS-17 panel is used, ensure it is visible from the air. At night, an inverted Y is used to designate the aircraft touchdown point. However, this may not be visible from the air. LZs should have a far recognition signal, such as a swinging chemlight or strobe light for easier locating.

3. Communications. Maintaining air-to-ground communications between the aircraft and the LZ will make movement times faster and assist the aircraft in locating the LZ.

4. Capacity. LZ selection is based on the number and type of aircraft that will be used for the CASEVAC operation. The LZ size will determine the number of aircraft that can be landed at one time to load casualties.

5. Obstacles. LZs should be free of obstacles such as cables, wires, antennas, large rocks, excessive slope, and large ruts making the location unsuitable. Obstacles that cannot be cleared from the location should be marked. If communications are maintained with the aircrew, LZ hazard advisories should be provided to the crews.

5.5.4.4 Landing Zone Criteria

Small unit leaders should be proficient in selecting and marking pickup zones (PZs)/LZs and in providing terminal guidance to aircraft. Each helicopter requires a different size PZ/LZ, and each area needs to be on level ground. Lighting conditions affect the size of the LZ for each helicopter: daylight zones should be 100 feet larger than the diameter of aircraft rotor blades and night zones should be 150 feet larger than the diameter of aircraft rotor blades.

There are three major considerations in evaluating the landing area:

1. The height of obstacles determines the approach angle. The higher the obstacle, the larger the area required for the helicopter to land. When tactically feasible and the aircraft is properly equipped, the only option is a hoist operation. A hoist operation takes longer to accomplish, and the aircraft is a more exposed target.

2. Clear debris and obstacles for a 50-meter radius of the LZ. Ensuring LZs in a combat environment are clear of debris within a 50-meter radius may not be possible. Helicopters produce high winds causing rotor washed debris to be thrown, injuring personnel and damaging equipment. Additional safety precautions for ground personnel include:

   a. Protecting eyes and patients from flying debris.

   b. Remaining clear of helicopter rotor blades and the tail rotor at all times.

   c. Exercising extreme caution on a sloped LZ because it may be difficult to see the spinning blades. Approaching from the upslope side could result in decapitation.

WARNING

Failure to observe safety precautions may result in injury or death.

3. Increased wind and the loss of wind affect helicopter power. Corpsmen must consider weather/wind factors that affect aircraft performance to achieve successful patient evacuation missions.

   a. A helicopter's hover ceilings are lower on a hot day than for a helicopter with the same gross weight and power settings on a day with standard temperatures.

   b. More casualties can be loaded on-board helicopters at higher altitudes with higher aircraft gross weights when the temperature is cool.

   c. Wind is a major factor in improving lift performance when considered with other factors, such as enemy positions and smoke drift, in accomplishing a successful patient evacuation. Understanding terrain wind flows enables corpsmen to:

      (1) Select the best LZ.

      (2) Anticipate safer helicopter approach/departure routes.

      (3) Anticipate the impact of LZ obstacles, such as tall trees, tall buildings, and power lines.

      (4) Provide valuable wind direction/estimated velocity information to aircrews.

   d. There are two major considerations in cold-weather patient evacuation operations:

      (1) Restricted visibility from blowing snow (whiteout) during helicopter landings

         (a) Improve restricted visibility by using smoke grenades or other objects distinguishable in color (pine boughs, painted jerry cans, or emergency kit) placed or planted as a reference point in the LZ. Smoke will aid in determining wind direction and speed. Do not use white smoke unless it is the only smoke available.

         (b) To prevent snow blindness and to protect the eyes from rotor-wash-caused debris, colored glasses or goggle inserts should be worn.

      (2) The adverse effect of cold temperatures (windchill) on the casualties and ground personnel loading casualties.

   e. Hot-weather patient evacuation operations may cause reduced power available in the aircraft, limiting the capability to hover out of ground effect. Hovering straight up and down may require a larger LZ. Flight crews may have restricted visibility (in desert areas) from blowing sand (brownout) near the point of touchdown and should wear goggles or glasses to prevent eye injuries.

For more information on landing zones, refer to MCWP 3-11.4, Helicopterborne Operations.

5.5.4.5 Landing Zone Procedures

1. Daylight landing procedures:

   a. Determine the LZ marking method, such as smoke or panel method.

   b. Do not use smoke until requested by aircrew. The enemy may launch the same-colored smoke and confuse pilots of the correct LZ location.

   c. Ensure dayglow panel markers (VS-17) are well secured to the ground when used to identify the LZ. Securing the markers to the ground will prevent them from being blown into the rotor system of the helicopter.

2. Night landing procedures:

   a. Maintain light discipline at night. Helicopter pilots and crew require the use of night-vision equipment.

   b. Turn on only the lights required to mark the LZ. Additional lighting requirements are directed by the helicopter crew.

   c. Vehicle headlights may be used to light the LZ when directed by the pilot. In peacetime and in exercise environments, vehicle headlight use is possible before CASEVAC or MEDEVAC arrives to aid the flight crew in locating the LZ. Ensure the headlights cast a glow on the anticipated touchdown point of the LZ to prevent blinding the pilots. Ensure the vehicles do not obstruct the LZ.

   d. Do not use smoke unless requested by the aircrew.

   e. Use chemlights to mark the boundaries of the LZ and any obstacles that may impair a safe landing.

5.5.4.6 Prepare and Load Casualties

1. Protecting casualties.

   a. Aircraft safety considerations. The litter and ambulatory casualties, the unit representative going with the casualties in peacetime, and those associated with loading casualties must be protected from the effects of the rotor blades, engine exhaust, and engine noise.

   b. Loading and unloading instructions. Most directions in loading casualties will be given by hand signals so roles should be established and understood before aircraft arrival. The corpsman should direct Marines tasked with loading casualties to protect themselves and the casualties prior to the arrival of the aircraft for the following reasons: it is quieter (unless taking fire), instructions can be heard and understood, and there is no time to accomplish this once the aircraft is on the deck. Aircraft present a large target in an LZ.

   c. Chill factor. Human efficiency is reduced as temperature drops and reduced sharply as temperature drops below -18 °C (0 °F). The human body is continually producing heat internally and losing it externally to the environment. Wind increases this heat loss particularly on exposed flesh. If the ambient air temperature is below freezing, the wind velocity removes heat from the body surface more rapidly than it can be replaced, and frostbite may occur. Ground personnel, casualties exposed to rotor wash, or flight crew at open hatches are particularly susceptible. Clothing or materiel which stops or reduces the wind gives a degree of protection to the covered area. Wet clothing has a reduced insulating value and results in heat loss nearly equal to that of exposed flesh. A person's skin (including casualties') shall not be exposed for any length of time under the rotor blast of a helicopter when in an arctic climate. Exposed skin may freeze in as little as 30 seconds.

    d. Aircraft exhaust hazard/ear protection zone areas. Corpsmen should be aware of aircraft engine exhaust hazards and ear protection zone areas to minimize casualty exposure.

2. Approaching the aircraft.

    a. Keep vehicles, nonessential personnel, and animals clear of the helicopter unless instructed by the aircrew.

    b. Never approach the helicopter unless directed by the aircrew. Medical personnel, if on board, will come to the patient unless under fire.

    c. Keep the area around the casualties clear to allow the corpsman to work more efficiently.

    d. Send a unit representative to secure personal belongings when the patient is admitted to the hospital. This will not occur in combat.

    e. Ensure the casualties are well protected from the elements, have received medical treatment, and have adequate IV fluid (if required). Medical tags should be properly filled out and well secured to prevent loss due to rotor or prop wash.

3. Requesting unit's responsibility. A patient evacuation request places the following responsibilities on the requesting unit:

    a. Ensure tactical situation permits evacuation.

    b. Ensure casualties and casualty information are ready when the request is submitted.

    c. Provide an English-speaking representative at the pickup site when evacuation is requested for non-US personnel.

    d. Receive backhauled medical supplies.

    e. Move casualties to the safest aircraft approach/departure point.

    f. Ensure ground personnel are familiar with principles of helicopter operations.

5.5.4.7 Planning Backhaul of Casualties During Vertical Assault Operations

During vertical assault operations, the MAGTF and ACE staffs plan for the use of lifting aircraft to backhaul casualties from the LZ. The MAGTF commander plans for support from CASEVAC and MEDEVAC aircraft. Flying CASEVAC aircraft during the air assault may conflict with the ongoing operation. The staff will plan for CASEVAC operations by the assaulting aircraft.

On air assaults with multiple lifts, the staff uses the lifting aircraft to pick up casualties during successive lifts. On single-lift air assaults, aircraft are designated to remain on standby for CASEVAC operations, usually at central forward arming and refueling points (FARPs), such as the LZ or an established holding area. The backhaul of casualties on a vertical assault is a critical mission for the utility helicopters and requires detailed planning.

The MAGTF command element (CE) and major subordinate command representatives must be involved in the planning stages of the air assault. If the commander's intent is to backhaul casualties, the planning must include the following considerations:

1. Casualty locations. The assault unit commander should designate an LZ to receive casualties, which facilitates rapid movement and minimizes aircraft LZ ground time. Members of the air assault task force should know the designated casualty point location upon arrival. This will allow focus on the casualty point and ground personnel will be prepared to accept casualties.

2. Signaling. Night operations provide a challenge for casualty backhaul operations. Evacuation planners should use light signals to indicate that aircraft arriving at the LZ should prepare to accept casualties.

3. Communications. Communications on a predesignated radio network can alert the flight to backhaul casualties from the LZ.

4. Designated area for dropping off casualties. The assault unit commander must determine where to transport casualties during a vertical assault and develop a plan for the use of CASEVAC helicopters. Casualties dropped off by lifting aircraft are loaded on CASEVAC aircraft for transportation to higher-level care facilities.

Considerations for selecting a casualty collection point (CCP) include the following:

a. Select a secure site with medical personnel ready to accept casualties. The site should be selected so that it does not interfere with a vertical assault.

b. Aircraft conducting casualty backhaul will separate from the serial at some point. The assault unit commander must be prepared to affect the bump plan if the aircraft carrying casualties does not return to the LZ for the next lift.

c. Aircraft arriving at the LZ full of casualties may cause confusion. Troops may be loading into the same aircraft from which casualties are unloading.

5.5.4.8 Air Requirements Plan

The MSOC will submit air evacuation designated standby aircraft requirements to the MLG ALO 72 hours in advance to ensure that helicopters are available for patient movement. MSOC SOPs consider the standby asset need based on the following parameters:

1. The greater the distance from the point of injury to first resuscitative care, the lower the survival rate of casualties requiring surgery, and the greater the dead of wounds (DOW) percentage.

2. The greater the distance from the point of injury to first resuscitative care, the less efficient are helicopter and ground transportation, and the more helicopters or ground vehicles are required.

3. The efficiency of helicopter litter casualty transport depends on the following factors:

a. Evacuation distance (time)

b. Maximum litter capacity of the helicopter

c. Range without refueling

d. Helicopter airspeed

e. Diversion distance (time) required for refueling

f. Number of aircraft requiring refueling, such as gunship escorts.

4. Staging helicopters, vehicles, and en route care teams forward reduces response times and facilitates optimal care while it utilizes lifts of opportunity, which increases effective transportation asset use.

5. The prevention of motion sickness, hypothermia, and other conditions that will be affected by low-altitude travel.

APPENDIX A

Patient Movement Task List

A.1 UNIVERSAL JOINT TASK LIST (UJTL)

1. SN 1.1.5, Determine Impact of Environmental Conditions on Strategic Mobility

2. SN 1.2.6, Conduct Redeployment or Retrograde of Personnel and Equipment from Theater

3. SN 1.2.8, Provide Global Patient Movement

4. SN 3.3.6, Determine National Residual Capabilities

5. SN 4.3.3, Coordinate Defense-wide Health Services

6. SN 6.6.4, Expand Health Service Support

7. SN 8.1, Support Other Nations or Groups

8. SN 8.2.3, Support Evacuation of Noncombatants from Theaters

9. ST 4.2.2, Coordinate Health Service Support

10. ST 4.2.2.2, Coordinate Patient Evacuation from Theater

11. ST 4.3.1, Establish and Coordinate Movement Services within Theater

12. OP 1.6, Conduct Patient Evacuation

13. OP 4.4.3, Provide for Health Services in the Joint Operations Area

14. OP 4.4.3.2, Manage Flow of Casualties in the Joint Operations Area

15. OP 4.4.3.3, Manage Health Services Resources in the Joint Operations Area

16. OP 4.4.5, Train Joint Forces and Personnel

17. OP 4.5.2, Supply Operational Forces

18. OP 4.5.3, Recommend Evacuation Policy and Procedures for the Joint Operations Area

19. OP 6.2.6, Conduct Evacuation of Noncombatants from the Joint Operations Area

20. TA 6.4, Conduct Noncombatant Evacuation

A.2 NAVY TACTICAL TASK LIST (NTTL)

1. NTA 1.2.8, Conduct Tactical Reconnaissance and Surveillance

2. NTA 4.7.8, Provide Humanitarian Support

3. NTA 4.8.1, Support Peace Operations

4. NTA 4.12, Provide Health Services

5. NTA 4.12.1, Perform Triage

6. NTA 4.12.3, Provide Surgical and Inpatient Care

7. NTA 4.12.5, Coordinate Patient Movement

8. NTA 4.12.7, Maintain Records

9. NTA 4.12.9, Train Medical and Non-medical Personnel

10. NTA 4.12.10, Provide Health Services in Support of Humanitarian and Civic Assistance

11. NTA 4.12.11, Provide Medical Staff Support

12. NTA 4.12.12, Perform Level II/III Medical Support

13. NTA 4.13, Conduct Recovery and Salvage

14. NTA 6.5.1, Provide Disaster Relief

A.3 MARINE CORPS TASK LIST (MCTL)

1. MCT 1.6.6.7, Conduct Humanitarian Assistance (HA) Operations

2. MCT 4.5, Provide Health Services

3. MCT 4.5.1, Conduct Health Maintenance

4. MCT 4.5.2, Perform Casualty Collection

5. MCT 4.5.3, Conduct Casualty Treatment

6. MCT 4.5.4, Conduct Temporary Casualty Holding

7. MCT 4.5.5, Conduct Casualty Evacuation

8. MCT 4.5.6, Conduct Mass Casualty Operations

9. MCT 4.6.1.7, Provide Civil Affairs Support

10. MCT 6.3, Perform Consequence Management

APPENDIX B

Health Service Support Capabilities

B.1 INTRODUCTION

The information contained in this appendix provides an overview of medical assets organic to Navy and Marine Corps forces.

For the Navy, additional information on HSS assets for specific unit/ship classes is found in NWP 4-02, Naval Expeditionary Health Service Support Afloat and Ashore, *and OPNAVINST 3501 (series),* Projected Operational Environment (POE) and Required Operational Capabilities (ROC).

For the Marine Corps, additional information on HSS assets is found in MCRP 5-12D, Organization of Marine Corps Forces; *MCWP 4-11.1,* Health Service Support Operations; *and MCRP 4-11.1E,* Health Service Support Field Reference Guide (draft).

At the joint level, for guidance on joint patient movement refer to JP 4-02, Health Service Support.

B.2 NAVY FORCES AFLOAT

B.2.1 Carrier Strike Group

The CSG is a naval task force composed of an aircraft carrier (CV/CVN) and supporting combatant ships capable of conducting strike operations. The notional CSG elements are CV/CVNs, guided missile cruisers, destroyers, frigates, attack submarines, and replenishment ships. The mission of the CV/CVN is to operate offensively in a high-density, multithreat environment as an integral member of a CSG or expeditionary strike force, and to provide credible, sustained forward presence, conventional deterrence, and support aircraft attacks in sustained operations. CV/CVN capabilities and staffing are shown in Figure B-1.

B.2.2 Expeditionary Strike Group

The ESG is a tactical organization of surface and subsurface combatants, maritime aviation, and assault shipping to transport troops and their equipment for expeditionary operations. The notional ESG elements are an amphibious assault ship (LHD/LHA), amphibious transport docks, surface combatants (guided missile cruisers, destroyers, or frigates), and an attack submarine.

B.2.2.1 Amphibious Assault Ship

The mission of the LHD/LHA is to operate offensively in a high density, multithreat environment as an integral member of the amphibious strike force or group; function as primary landing ships for MEFs; and function as the CRTS when the FST is embarked. The CRTS requires the Health Services Augmentation Program (HSAP) augmentees to provide full expanded HSS capabilities. The LHD/LHA capabilities and staffing for the TARAWA and WASP class are shown in Figure B-2.

CV/CVN CAPABILITY	STAFFING
Operating Rooms	1
Intensive Care Unit Beds	3
Ward Beds	51
Ancillary Capabilities	Laboratory, x ray, pharmacy, preventive medicine, biomedical repair, aviation physical examinations, radiation health, spectacle fabrication, pyschology, physical therapy, and Substance Abuse Rehabilitation Program (SARP) screening
Complement (Ship's Company and Air Wing)	
Medical Corps	6*
Dental Corps	5
Nurse Corps	2
Medical Service Corps	5
Hospital Corpsmen	49**
* Includes embarked physicians	
** Includes two SARP counselors attached to the medical department	

Figure B-1. Aircraft Carrier Capabilities and Staffing

LHD/LHA CAPABILITY	SHIP/FST STAFFING		SHIP/FST/HSAP STAFFING	
Operating Rooms	1		4	
Intensive Care Unit Beds	3		15	
Ward Beds	12		45	
Ancillary Capabilities	Laboratory, x ray, pharmacy, preventive medicine, biomedical repair, aviation physical examination		Laboratory, x ray, pharmacy, preventive medicine, biomedical repair, aviation physical examination	
	SHIP	FST*		HSAP
Complement				
Medical Corps	2	3**		11
Dental Corps	1			1
Nurse Corps		3**		22
Medical Service Corps	1	1		1
Hospital Corpsmen	19	9		49
* The FST officer in charge can be 2XXX				
** Includes certified registered anesthesiologist or nurse anesthetist				

Figure B-2. Amphibious Assault Ship Capabilities and Staffing

B.2.2.2 Amphibious Transport Dock

The mission of the amphibious transport dock, or LPD, is to transport and land Marines and their equipment and supplies by embarked landing craft or amphibious vehicles augmented by helicopters. The LPD SAN ANTONIO class contains enhanced C2 features and a robust communications suite that improves its ability to support embarked landing forces, a MAGTF, and joint and friendly forces. It is equipped with operating rooms (ORs) and ward beds without the staffing capability. Figure B-3 shows LPD capabilities and staffing for the AUSTIN and the SAN ANTONIO classes.

B.2.2.3 Dock Landing Ship

The mission of the landing ship dock, or LSD, is to transport and land Marines, and their equipment and supplies either by embarked landing craft or amphibious vehicles augmented by helicopters, and to support amphibious operations including landings by way of landing craft air cushion. Figure B-4 lists LSD capabilities and staffing for the HARPERS FERRY and WHIDBEY ISLAND classes.

B.2.3 Submarine Tender

The mission of the submarine tender (AS) is to provide at-sea support capability. Figure B-5 lists submarine tender capabilities and staffing.

B.2.4 Surface Combatants

The surface combatant ships — cruiser, destroyer, and frigate— have limited HSS capabilities and staffing. Their ancillary capability consists of one basic laboratory. Hospital corpsmen are made up of one independent duty hospital corpsman and one junior hospital corpsman (HM).

LPD CAPABILITY	AUSTIN CLASS STAFFING	SAN ANTONIO CLASS STAFFING
Operating Rooms	0	1
Ward Beds	17	24
Ancillary Capabilities	Laboratory and x ray	Laboratory and x ray
Complement		
Medical Corps	1	1
Dental Corps	1	1
Hospital Corpsmen	9	15

Figure B-3. Amphibious Transport Dock Capabilities and Staffing

LSD CAPABILITY	STAFFING
Ward Beds (2 isolation beds)	8
Ancillary Capabilities	Laboratory and x ray
Complement	
Medical Corps	1
Dental Corps	1
Hospital Corpsmen	5

Figure B-4. Landing Ship Dock Capabilities and Staffing

AS CAPABILITY	STAFFING
Operating Rooms	2
Ward Beds	12
Ancillary Capabilities	Laboratory, x ray, and pharmacy
Complement	
Medical Corps	1
Dental Corps	3
Hospital Corpsmen	18

Figure B-5. Submarine Tender Capabilities and Staffing

B.2.5 Hospital Ship

Hospital ships (T-AHs) are operated by the Military Sealift Command and are designed to provide emergency, on-site care for US combatant forces deployed in war and other operations. The T-AHs provide a mobile, flexible, rapidly responsive afloat medical capability to acute medical and surgical care in support of ATF; Marine Corps, Army, and Air Force elements; forward-deployed Navy elements of the fleet; and fleet activities located in areas where hostilities may be imminent. The T-AHs also provide a full-service hospital asset for use by other government agencies involved in the support of disaster relief and humanitarian operations worldwide. HSS capabilities and staffing for the T-AHs are shown in Figure B-6.

T-AH CAPABILITY	STAFFING
Operating Rooms	12
Intensive Care Unit Beds	100 (includes 20 postsurgical recovery beds)
Intermediate Care Beds	400
Minimal Care Beds	500
Ancillary Capabilities	Laboratory, x ray, pharmacy, computerized tomography scanner, blood storage
Complement (staffing up to 1,000 beds)	
Medical Corps	66
Medical Service Corps	20
Nurse Corps	168
Hospital Corpsmen	698
Nonmedical Officers	14
Nonmedical Enlisted	244
Dental Corps	4

Figure B-6. Hospital Ship Capabilities and Staffing

B.3 NAVY FORCES ASHORE

NAVFOR ashore have been combined under the NECC, the functional command that centrally manages current and future readiness, resources, manning, training, and equipping of the Navy's expeditionary forces. There are HSS personnel and equipment organic to each NAVFOR ashore component. The range of medical capabilities includes first responder and FRC accomplished by a hospital corpsman and medical officers assigned to the unit, and by the establishment of a BAS when deployed. The organization of HSS consists of the SMO, the SMDR, a hospital corpsman, and litter bearers. The physicians serve at the group level in general medical officer and diving medical officer positions.

B.3.1 Senior Medical Officer

The unit's SMO is designated as the department head for the medical department. In addition to those duties prescribed by Navy Regulations for a head of department, the SMO is responsible, under the CO, for maintaining the health of all attached personnel, conducting inspections, and advising the CO with respect to health and sanitation affecting the command. The SMO is responsible for ensuring that all medical providers attached to the unit are properly credentialed and privileged and that they exercise only those clinical privileges that can be reasonably supported by the ship's medical capabilities. The SMO is responsible for all medical department materiel on board and will be in charge of the sick and injured. The SMO may be required to give medical support to other units, including training and oversight of all medical department personnel.

B.3.2 Senior Medical Department Representative

A senior hospital IDC serves in the absence of a medical officer, is designated the unit's SMDR, and functions as the unit's primary care provider. The IDC works for a physician preceptor. The SMDR assumes the technical medical responsibilities of a unit's medical officer as defined in Paragraph B.3.1, as qualifications allow. The SMDR is responsible to the CO for the following:

1. Care of the sick and injured

2. Sanitation and hygiene of the command

3. Health of personnel

4. Preparation of medical reports and records

5. Maintenance of medical supplies and equipment

6. Training of medical and nonmedical personnel.

B.3.3 Hospital Corpsman

Hospital corpsmen from each unit are responsible for the following:

1. Providing first aid for casualties

2. Preparing patients for evacuation

3. Ensuring preventive medicine is practiced

4. Making recommendations to the unit commanders concerning rigorous programs of field sanitation and personal hygiene

5. Providing immediate treatment of minor ailments.

B.3.4 Litter Bearer

A litter bearer group operates under the direction of the medical department. Litter bearers are Sailors assigned by the unit commander, not part of the battalion medical section. Early designation of litter bearers is essential for training in the proper techniques of casualty handling.

B.4 MARINE CORPS

The Marine Corps operating forces are organized into MAGTFs for conducting combat operations. The type of MAGTF HSS would be supporting is dictated by the contingency. The three types of MAGTFs are a Marine expeditionary unit (MEU), Marine expeditionary brigade (MEB), or a Marine expeditionary force (MEF).

Each MAGTF, regardless of size, is a combination of forces made up of the following four elements:

1. The command element (CE) has C2 of the MAGTF; personnel can be sourced from any of the supporting units.

2. The ground combat element (GCE) consists of MARDIV personnel.

3. An aviation combat element (ACE) consists of Marine aircraft wing (MAW) personnel.

4. The logistics combat element (LCE) consists of MLG personnel.

HSS personnel and equipment are organic to each MAGTF element. HSS elements are sized and equipped to support personnel and mission requirements when assigned to a MAGTF:

B.4.1 Command Element

The MEF CE medical staff consists of the MEF surgeon, MEF medical planner, MEF preventive medicine officer, MEB medical planner, operations chief, preventive medicine chief, and administrative chief. The MEF CE provides routine and emergency HSS by using its major subordinate command's HSS personnel.

The MLG CE medical staff consists of a group surgeon, a group aid station, and an HSSE. The group surgeon functions as a special staff officer advising the MLG commander on matters relating to the health of the MLG personnel. The group surgeon provides clinical oversight of the group aid station, which provides internal HSS to the MLG. The HSSE serves as the principal HSS planner for the MLG and coordinates the requirements for HSS and Class VIII A and B supplies required above the organic capabilities of the GCE and the ACE. The HSSO manages the HSSE and serves as the principal planner for the MLG.

B.4.2 Ground Combat Element

The GCE of a MAGTF is comprised of MARDIV units sized to the mission. A MARDIV is the GCE for a MEF, a Marine regimental landing team (RLT) is the GCE for a MEB, and a Marine BLT is the GCE for an MEU.

The division CE medical staff consists of the division surgeon, a psychiatrist, a medical administrative officer, an environmental health officer, and enlisted staff to provide administrative support, training, and senior enlisted leadership to all subordinate medical personnel within the division. The division surgeon functions as a special staff officer who advises the division commander on all matters relating to the health of the division, including HSS requirements and the allocation of medical resources.

B.4.2.1 Regimental Aid Station

The regimental aid station (RAS) contains all medical support organic to the regimental HQ company. Because there is only one medical officer and three hospital corpsmen, the RAS is unable to meet the same level of casualty flow as a BAS, which has more medical personnel. The RAS is augmented by its own battalion personnel or from nondeploying regiments within the division. It can be reinforced by an STP or FRSS, as indicated in Annex Q of the OPLAN or OPORD. The mission of the RAS is to:

1. Coordinate and support medical care to the rifle battalions, attached units, and company HQ.

2. Coordinate CASEVAC from the battalions and attached units to the appropriate next level of medical care.

3. Provide limited medical care to the personnel of company HQ.

4. Consolidate casualty and illness reports from attached units and forward them to the regimental command post and to HHQ. The regimental HQ medical staff consists of the regimental surgeon, the regimental senior chief hospital corpsman, the chief hospital corpsman preventive medicine technician, and the hospital corpsman third class.

    a. The regimental surgeon is a special staff officer, a planner, organizer, teacher, supervisor, and advisor in addition to duties in patient treatment. The regimental surgeon advises the regimental commander and staff on all matters pertaining to the health of the regiment and performs other duties as directed by the regimental commander. The surgeon directs the activities of the RAS.

    b. The regimental senior chief hospital corpsman is the administrative and chief medical assistant to the regimental surgeon.

    c. The chief hospital corpsman preventive medicine technician advises the regimental surgeon and the regimental commander on preventive medicine issues.

    d. The hospital corpsman third class serves as ambulance driver, radio communicator and medical supply technician for the RAS, and maintains medical and dental records of personnel attached to company HQ.

B.4.2.2 Battalion Aid Station

The BAS is staffed by the following personnel:

1. Medical staff. The medical staff of an infantry battalion or battalion medical platoon consists of 2 medical officers, 65 hospital corpsmen, and 51 organic and 13 HSAP billets.

    a. Battalion surgeon. One medical officer in an infantry battalion is designated as the battalion surgeon, a special staff officer who advises the battalion commander on matters pertaining to the health of the battalion. The battalion surgeon supervises patient treatment, plans, organizes, trains the battalion medical staff, and performs other duties as directed by the battalion commander.

    b. Assistant battalion surgeon. The second medical officer in an infantry battalion is designated as the assistant battalion surgeon. Duties include to direct, manage, and supervise the operation of the BASs and additional duties as directed by the battalion surgeon.

    c. Aid station. The aid station, consisting of 21 of the 65 hospital corpsmen in an infantry battalion, is assigned to the BAS under the supervision of the assistant battalion surgeon. This group is capable of splitting into two sections to operate two separate BASs. The battalion surgeon heads the second aid station.

    d. Company medical teams. The remaining 44 hospital corpsmen assigned to the battalion medical platoon are divided into 4 groups called company medical teams. The four medical teams are assigned to the weapons company with one assigned to each of the three rifle companies of an infantry battalion.

The team is responsible for the following:

(1) Provides first aid for casualties

(2) Prepares patients for evacuation

(3) Ensures preventive medicine is practiced

(4) Makes recommendations to the unit commanders concerning rigorous programs of field sanitation and personal hygiene

(5) Provides immediate treatment of minor ailments.

e. Company corpsman. The senior hospital corpsman from each company medical team is designated as the company corpsman and is assigned to the company HQ. The remaining corpsmen are designated platoon corpsmen.

Note

Field ambulance service and CASEVAC procedures are contained in the battalion SOP or in the administrative/logistics order. Emergency casualty evacuation, special medical assistance, and other medical matters not specifically covered in battalion SOPs or administrative/logistics orders are requested through the S-4 (logistics) officer.

f. Litter bearer group. Early designation of litter bearers is essential for training in the proper techniques of casualty handling. A litter bearer group operates under the supervision of the battalion surgeon. Litter bearers are Marines assigned by the battalion or regimental commander not part of the battalion medical section.

2. Nonmedical personnel. While not part of the RAS, BAS, or other MTF, several nonmedical personnel are required for the provision of medical services. The senior Marine commander assigns the duties for handling the provision of medical services, which temporarily operates under the supervision of the organization senior surgeon. The following specific nonmedical personnel perform medical service duties:

a. Litter bearers. Litter bearers are vital for the survival of the casualty, maintenance of good morale, and preventing loss of firepower to the assaulting platoons and companies. Early designation of litter bearers is essential for proper training in casualty handling procedures.

b. Ambulance drivers. Two ambulance drivers from the motor transport section will be assigned during operations and exercises. This allows the medical personnel to be used most efficiently in the performance of medical duties. Hospital corpsmen are also trained to drive vehicles.

c. Armorers/Security. Security personnel must search and disarm all patients brought to the MTF before being admitted. Armorers collect and secure confiscated weapons. Enemy prisoners of war (EPWs) must be guarded while in the MTF. Medical personnel attending to the sick and wounded must not be used for securing weapons or guarding prisoners.

d. CBRN patient decontamination personnel. All patients must be decontaminated before entering the MTF. Nonmedical personnel must be identified to assist in the decontamination of patients. There are insufficient medical personnel available to do both emergency medical treatment and patient decontamination. These personnel are trained in patient decontamination procedures in advance of the OPORD.

e. Religious personnel. A chaplain and religious programs specialist are at the MTF when casualties are being received.

B.4.3 Aviation Combat Element

The ACE of a MAGTF is comprised of MAW units (fixed-wing and/or rotary-wing) to support the mission. A MAW is the ACE for a MEF; a Marine aircraft group (MAG) is the ACE for a MEB; and a Marine aircraft squadron/or composite squadron is the ACE for an MEU. HSS personnel are assigned to the primary subordinate organizations in the MAW. The Marine wing support group (MWSG) and Marine wing support squadron (MWSS) provide aid station capability for expeditionary airfield operations.

The wing CE medical staff consists of the wing medical officer or wing surgeon, a medical administrative officer, an environmental health officer, an industrial hygienist, and enlisted personnel. The wing medical officer or wing surgeon functions as a special staff officer, advising the wing commander on all matters relating to the health of the wing, including the development of medical policies for the wing, training of medical and nonmedical personnel, HSS requirements, and allocation of medical resources. The remainder of the wing surgeon's staff is responsible for medical planning, logistics, coordination of administrative functions, maintenance of records, and personnel administration.

A group medical section for each MAG HQ consists of a medical officer and two hospital corpsmen. The MAG medical officer carries out the wing surgeon's policies, performs duties in support of the MAG personnel, and is a special advisor to the MAG commander. The MWSG includes 4 MWSSs with organic (from the unit) medical assets consisting of 2 medical officers, 31 to 32 hospital corpsmen, and the equipment and supplies to establish a squadron aid station. The MWSS aid station is capable of providing routine sick call; aviation medicine; preventive medicine; and laboratory, radiology and pharmacy services.

Each flying squadron within a MAG has a medical section consisting of a flight surgeon and a number of hospital corpsmen depending on squadron type. The squadron medical section provides a pool of trained in-flight corpsmen for CASEVAC missions and conducts routine sick call and other aviation medical functions. In order to centralize organization and support, squadron medical personnel normally work in conjunction with the MWSS aid station.

B.4.4 Logistics Combat Element

The LCE is a core element of the MAGTF and is responsible for the combat service support necessary to accomplish the MAGTF mission. LCEs are further defined in the four types of MAGTFs. The LCE for a MEF is a MLG, the LCE for a MEB is a combat logistics regiment (CLR), and the LCE for an MEU is a CLB. The mission of LCE HSS is to sustain the fighting ability of the MAGTF, to return as many casualties to duty as soon as possible, and to stabilize and prepare for evacuation of casualties whose length of stay is expected to exceed the MAGTF evacuation policy. This mission is accomplished through the operation of a BES and/or HES organized to provide emergency treatment, to collect casualty evacuation, and to provide preventive medicine services.

B.4.5 Medical Battalion

The medical battalion is the primary source of HSS above the RAS/BAS and provides direct and general medical support to the MEF. The medical battalion's mission is to perform emergency medical and surgical procedures that, if not performed, could lead to death or loss of limb or body function. The battalion structure has 260 holding beds and 9 operating suites and is made up of a headquarters and service (H&S) company and 3 surgical companies. The H&S company contains 8 STPs with 10 patient holding beds. Each surgical company contains 60 beds and 3 operating suites (6 tables). A dental detachment may augment each surgical company to provide dental treatment and medical support as needed.

Each medical battalion has FRSS equipment sets. The FRSS is capable of providing a spectrum of trauma care ranging from triage, advance trauma life support, and stabilization through salvage surgical procedures. The team is composed of eight personnel. FRSS staffing is constrained to the existing medical battalion table of organization. The FRSS is task-organized using manpower from the surgical companies.

Note

> The battalion structure of 260 holding beds applies to 1st and 2nd medical battalions only. The 3rd and 4th medical battalions have 180 holding beds, 2 surgical companies, and 6 STPs.

The medical battalion is organized to execute HSS functions in support of the MEF. It is structured to facilitate task organization for operations conducted by the battalion in support of the MEF or any combination of smaller MAGTFs operating in widely separated geographical areas. The medical battalion may be task-organized to provide STPs, FRSSs, and en route care.

For further information about the FRSS, refer to MCRP 4-11.1E, Health Service Support Field Reference Guide (draft).

B.4.6 Headquarters and Service Company, Medical Battalion

The H&S company provides C2 and support functions for the medical battalion. It collects, clears, and evacuates casualties from supported MEF elements through the STPs and provides comprehensive preventive medical services to all supported units. The H&S company may be employed in a single or two separate combat service support areas (CSSAs) to provide C2 facilities and administrative support for the battalion.

The H&S company plans, coordinates, and supervises the command support functions for the battalion. It facilitates task organization for operations conducted by the battalion in support of MAGTF operations. The H&S company comprises several sections: administration and personnel, intelligence and operations, logistics, communications, chaplain, preventive medicine, and STPs.

B.4.6.1 Shock Trauma Platoons

The STP is a mobile medical support element with the medical battalion and is the first MTF of the MAGTF in support of the BAS. The STP provides direct medical support to the MEF, including collecting, clearing, and evacuating casualties from supported MEF elements, and MTFs for resuscitative treatment care and temporary holding of casualties. The STP provides direct support to the MEF, MEB, or any combination of smaller MAGTFs. Although a degree of mobility is sacrificed in providing a patient treatment facility, the STP must maintain the capability to evacuate casualties and move in support of BASs and the MAGTF elements it serves.

The methods by which this facility is established, displaced, and relocated must keep pace with the mobility and flexibility demanded by MAGTF operations. The platoon is capable of limited organic supply support to receive, temporarily hold, account for, and issue Class VIII supplies. It serves as a limited emergency resupply source for medical materiel for supported medical units. All other nonmedical supply support is provided by the H&S company of the medical battalion. Medical supply support is provided by the medical logistics company.

1. The STP consists of a stabilization section and a collecting and evacuation section.

    a. Stabilization section. The STP stabilization section is highly mobile and provides advance trauma life support, the nucleus for a ten flow through cot (litter) facility, and evacuation stations for emergency treatment, triage, and ambulance transfer points.

The section consists of the following staff:

(1) Two emergency medical officers

(2) One physician's assistant

(3) One independent duty corpsman

(4) Seven field medical technicians.

b. Collecting and evacuation section. The STP collecting and evacuation section collects and transfers casualties and provides advance trauma life support with supporting staff and transporting equipment.

(1) Staffing for the collecting and evacuation section includes:

(a) One nurse corps officer

(b) One IDC

(c) Six field medical technicians

(d) Six Marine motor vehicle operators

(e) One radio operator.

(2) Vehicle transporting equipment for the collecting and evacuation section includes:

(a) One HMMWV

(b) Two tactical ambulances (M997 A2) for collecting casualties from the next forward medical support echelon

(c) Two 7-ton trucks (MK 23) with an M105 trailer to move STP personnel and equipment.

2. In Operation IRAQI FREEDOM (OIF), STPs were combined with FRSSs to provide triage and pre-/postoperative care. STPs can be combined or collocated to:

a. Increase capabilities and care provided to Marines.

b. Relieve a BAS of patients, allowing the BAS to follow in trace of its supported element.

c. Act as the advance element for the location of a surgical company.

d. Function as part of a mobile combat logistics company (CLC).

3. The STPs provide communications and patient movement support to the FRSSs.

B.4.6.2 Surgical Company, Medical Battalion

The company provides general HSS to the MEF, including MTFs for medical and surgical care and temporary casualty holding. A surgical company is structured to facilitate task-organization for operations conducted by the battalion in support of the MEB, MEF, or any combination of MAGTFs. The surgical company design allows a high degree of deployment mobility and flexibility. It can be divided into smaller elements (sections) to task-organize support for a deploying platoon or section in the assault echelon and use the remaining capability for the assault follow-on echelon (AFOE) shipping. In a displacement and relocation evolution, platoons and sections can be deployed in a leapfrog fashion to provide maximum continuity of patient care. A surgical section can augment the medical facility of an MWSS, bringing surgical capability to that facility. The surgical company is suited for augmenting an STP when operational conditions permit. Each surgical company consists of the following platoons:

1. HQ platoon

2. Triage/evacuation platoon

3. Surgical platoon with 3 surgical sections (3 operating suites or 6 tables)

4. Holding platoon with 3 ward sections (20 beds each)

5. Combat stress platoon

6. Ancillary service platoon with two laboratory sections and two x-ray sections.

Although a fully deployed surgical company is best suited for a general support role from a location less likely to require displacement and relocation, the surgical company structure and organization lends itself to dividing into independent elements for deployment to provide direct support to operating forces through the use of STPs. The triage/evacuation platoon of a surgical company can be deployed with the assault echelon of a combat force while the holding and surgical platoons are placed in the assault follow-on echelon. Once ashore, the remaining surgical company units join the triage/evacuation platoon that can establish in a different location.

B.4.6.3 Dental Battalion

The dental battalion of the MLG provides maintenance and emergency dental care and specialized care of casualties with maxillofacial injuries. The battalion is composed of approximately 70 dental corps officers, 2 MSC officers, and 125 hospital corpsmen. The dental battalion includes an H&S company and three dental companies.

Each dental company is capable of providing general support dental health care to the major subordinate elements of the MEF including emergency dental treatment and specialty disciplines with the exception of maxillofacial surgery. Task-organized dental support detachments can be employed to support any element of the MEF or to reinforce other dental and/or medical units. A dental detachment may be attached to each surgical company of the MLG and wing aid stations. The detachment is equipped and staffed to provide for routine dental care but may be used to assist medical personnel in the event of mass casualties.

B.5 THEATER SUPPORT

B.5.1 Theater Patient Movement Requirements Center

The TPMRC is a joint activity assigned to the COCOMs that provide medical regulating, clinical validation, patient ITV, patient movement planning, and execution support to respective theaters. The TPMRCs communicate intratheater patient movement requirements with respective air mobility operations command centers and Service components responsible for executing the mission. TPMRCs generate operational AE plans for the theater and coordinate patient regulating and movement with supporting activities, AE elements, and MTF activities to ensure seamless patient movement and ITV. TPMRCs coordinate intertheater AE requirements with USTRANSCOM, GPRMC, and TACC for planning, execution, and integration with theater patient movement systems.

B.5.2 Patient Movement Item System

The PMI system supports patient ITV, exchange of in-kind PMIs without degrading medical capabilities, and recycling of PMIs. The originating MTF is responsible for notifying the PMRC for special medical equipment needs for patient transport. PMIs are medical equipment and durable supplies that must be available to support the patient, including ventilators, litters, patient monitors, and pulse oximeters. The Air Force CCDR is responsible for the establishment of theater PMI centers and cells. The PMIs accompany a patient throughout the chain of movement, from the originating MTF to the destination MTF, whether it is an intratheater or intertheater transfer. PMI centers are established to support worldwide theater requirements.

PMI centers will be located at aerial ports of embarkation and/or debarkation within CONUS and outside the continental United States (OCONUS) to match AE support plans. The PMI centers and cells will receive, refurbish, redistribute, and return items collected from MTFs. Refurbishing includes technical inspection, calibration, repair, and replenishment of expendable supplies to maintain a three-day level of supplies. At the time, an MTF initiates a PMR requiring PMIs, the PMI center and/or cell will initiate action for the exchange of in-kind PMIs. Equipment sent with evacuated patients or transferred patients should be documented on the EMF's equipment records for auditing and accountability in accordance with the applicable NAVSUP, BUMED, or NAVFAC instructions.

B.5.3 Strategic Aeromedical Evacuation

USTRANSCOM is responsible for intertheater/strategic evacuation. Strategic AE capabilities may consist of dedicated and/or opportune aircraft equipped and medically staffed for patient evacuation. The Air Force is the lead Service for strategic AE. Expeditionary HSS units must coordinate AE with an AELT and an aeromedical staging facility (ASF) or MASF. These are medical facilities established by the Air Force in theater for the purpose of coordinating entry of patients into the theater AE system and temporarily holding patients prior to strategic AE. Patients will be transported to these facilities for evacuation. Upon request, the Air Force will assign an AELT to a hospital ship. The AELT will provide coordination services for strategic AE.

B.5.4 Evacuation Requests

Various communication forms and formats such as voice, radio, and message are used by each Service to request initial evacuation. To request further evacuation, a PMR is submitted by the medical facility patient administration or medical regulating office to the appropriate PMRC. The PMRC evaluates the request for necessity, acuity, eligibility, priority, and mode. PMRs are submitted through USTRANSCOM regulating and C2 evacuation system for ITV. PMRs may be submitted by facsimile, voice telephone, radio and/or satellite communications, using a standard PMR worksheet, when USTRANSCOM's regulating and C2 evacuation system is inaccessible. Patient information items required to request patient movement are determined by the PMRC and depend on the operational environment.

Intertheater operations are global. They serve the transportation needs of the combatant command outside the AOR and support the conduct of operations within the AOR. USTRANSCOM directs policies and procedures for intertheater patient movement and identifies transport resources. Currently, intertheater patient movement is conducted using airlift assets as long evacuation distances may preclude other modes of patient movement in supporting rapid evacuation out of the COCOM AOR. Patients are most likely to enter the intertheater system from a theater hospitalization capability for movement to a definitive care capability outside the theater of operations or eventually to CONUS. Intertheater patient movement requires a coordinated effort among the Services or HN MTFs, responsible PMRCs, GPMRCs, and transportation agencies.

APPENDIX C

Reports

C.1 SUBMITTING REPORTS

All reports may be transmitted by SIPRNET e-mail or as voice reports on secure field telephone, secure iridium phone, or over the MEDREGNET. General guidelines, OPLANs, OPORDs, and HHQ policy provide criteria for submitting reports.

C.1.1 Afloat Report

Afloat reports are submitted to the strike group surgeon, EMF reporting senior or higher authority, with a copy to the MRT.

C.1.2 Ashore Report

The ashore report is submitted to the MSOC or higher authority with a copy to the PET. The MSOC forwards the report to all major subordinate commands, and the MEF posts them to the SIPRNET Web page.

C.2 MEDICAL SITUATION REPORT

The medical situation report, submitted daily, provides a common operating picture on the status of HSS assets of Navy and Marine Corps operating forces. (See Paragraphs C.4 through C.6 and Figures C-1 through C-4 for report formats and report/request voice templates.)

C.3 ADMISSIONS REPORT

MTFs with holding beds and cots submit an admission report to HQ daily that identifies patients admitted to the MTF within a 24-hour period. Depending on the volume of patients, the requirement to submit this report may change to every 12 hours.

C.4 MEDICAL JOINING REPORT

MTFs submit a medical joining report when they become operational. The following is an example of a joining report:

FM: [NAME OF UNIT]

TO: NAVY [STRIKE GROUP/EMF REPORTING SENIOR]
       MARINE CORPS [MSOC]

INFO: NAVY [MRT]
       MARINE CORPS [PET/MEF]

SUBJ: MEDICAL JOINING REPORT

REF: (A) NTTP 4-02.2M

RMKS/1. PER THE REFERENCES, THE MEDICAL JOINING REPORT FOR THE [NAME OF UNIT] IS SUBMITTED.

2. NUMBER OF DEDICATED OPERATING ROOMS

3. NUMBER OF OTHER OPERATING AREAS EQUIPPED WITH SUITABLE EQUIPMENT NEEDED FOR THE PERFORMANCE OF BASIC SURGICAL PROCEDURES

4. NUMBER OF FIXED X-RAY MACHINES

5. NUMBER OF PORTABLE X-RAY MACHINES

6. NUMBER OF REFRIGERATORS SUITABLE FOR WHOLE BLOOD STORAGE/TOTAL CAPACITY OF REFRIGERATORS IN BLOOD UNITS

7. NUMBER OF BLOOD UNITS ON HAND LISTED BY ABO/RH TYPES

8. NUMBER OF ICU BEDS AVAILABLE

9. NUMBER OF OTHER BEDS AVAILABLE

10. NUMBER OF OVERFLOW BEDS SUITABLE FOR CASUALTY CARE

C.5 FACILITIES SPOT STATUS REPORT AND VOICE TEMPLATE

C.5.1 Facilities Spot Status Report

Upon request of higher authority, MTFs submit a facilities spot status report to identify changes and ensure that HHQ has the most current information for making patient movement decisions. The following is an example of a facilities spot status report:

FM: [NAME OF UNIT]

TO: NAVY [STRIKE GROUP/EMF REPORTING SENIOR]
        MARINE CORPS [MSOC]

INFO: NAVY [MRT]
        MARINE CORPS [PET/MEF]

SUBJ: FACILITIES SPOT STATUS REPORT AS OF [DTG]

REF: (A) NTTP 4-02.2M

RMKS/1. PER THE REFERENCES, THE FACILITIES SPOT STATUS REPORT FOR THE [NAME OF UNIT] IS SUBMITTED.

ALPHA: [OPERATING BEDS]

BRAVO: [BEDS OCCUPIED]

CHARLIE: [MAJOR ORS]

CHARLIE ONE: [PATIENT BACKLOG]

CHARLIE TWO: [HOURS BACKLOG]

DELTA: [MINOR OPERATING ROOMS]

DELTA ONE: [PATIENT BACKLOG]

DELTA TWO: [HOURS BACKLOG]

ECHO: [PATIENTS FOR LATERAL TRANSFER]

FOXTROT: [PATIENTS FOR EVACUATION OUT OF AOR]

GOLF: [REMARKS].

NOTES: Lines ECHO and FOXTROT must be coded by patient type:

Burn (SB)

Cardio-Thoracic (SSC)

Gen Surgery (SS)

Medical (MM)

Neurosurgery (SSN)

OB/GYN (SG)

Ophthalmology (SSO)

Oral/Maxillofacial (SSM)

Orthopedic (SO)

Pediatric (MC)

Psychiatric (MP)

Spinal Cord (SC)

Thoracic (SSC)

Urology (SSU)

C.5.2 Voice Template for Facilities Spot Status Report

"[Addressee], this is [Originator]. Over."

"[Originator], this is [Addressee]. Over."

"This is [Originator]. Request spot status report. Over."

"Roger. Status report for [Addressee] follows. Break."

[DTG]: _____

[UNIT CALL SIGN]: _____

LINE ALPHA [OPERATIONAL BEDS]: _____

LINE BRAVO [BEDS OCCUPIED]: _____

LINE CHARLIE ONE [MAJOR SURG BACKLOG # PATIENTS]: _____

LINE CHARLIE TWO: [MAJOR SURG BACKLOG # HOURS]: _____

DELTA ONE [MINOR SURG BACKLOG # PATIENTS]: _____

DELTA TWO: [MINOR SURG BACKLOG # HOURS]: _____

ECHO: [PATIENTS FOR LATERAL TRANSFER]: _____

FOXTROT: [PATIENTS FOR EVAC OUT OF AOR]: _____

GOLF: [REMARKS]

_____

_____

____

"HOW COPY. OVER."

FACILITIES SPOT STATUS REPORT

FM: (MTF)
TO: (MRCO)

FACILITIES SPOT STATUS REPORT AS OF (DTG)
SPOT STATUS REPORT AS OF (DTG)
ALPHA: (OPERATING BEDS)

BRAVO: (BEDS OCCUPIED)

CHARLIE: (MAJOR ORS)
               CHARLIE ONE: (PATIENT BACKLOG)
               CHARLIE TWO: (HOURS BACKLOG)

DELTA: (MINOR ORS)
               DELTA ONE: (PATIENT BACKLOG)
               DELTA TWO: (HOURS BACKLOG)

ECHO: (PATIENTS FOR LATERAL TRANSFER)

FOXTROT: (PATIENTS FOR EVAC OUT OF AOR)
               OUT OF AOA)
GOLF: (REMARKS)

NOTES:

1. OMIT LINES NOT CHANGED FROM PREVIOUS REPORT. INITIAL REPORT MUST INCLUDE ALL LINES.

2. LINES E AND F MUST BE CODED.

Figure C-1. Facilities Spot Status Report

C.6 BLOOD STATUS REPORT/REQUEST

BLOOD STATUS REPORT/REQUEST

FM: (UNIT)
TO: (CATF/CLF)
SUBJ: BLOOD STATUS REPORT/REQUEST

1. PASS TO BLOOD PROGRAM OFFICER.
PROGRAM OFFICER.

(CODE LINE)	(ITEM)	(NOTE)
ALPHA ONE:	(DTG AT END OF REPORTING PERIOD)	2
ALPHA TWO:	(UNIT/FACILITY REPORTING)	
ALPHA THREE:	(UNIT LOCATION IF CHANGED)	1, 6
BRAVO ONE:	(NUMBER OF UNITS ON HAND)	1, 3
BRAVO TWO:	(EXPIRATION DATE BY ABO/RH OF LATEST)	1, 3
CHARLIE ONE:	(TOTAL UNITS TRANSFUSED DURING PERIOD)	1
CHARLIE TWO:	(TOTAL UNITS EXPENDED DURING PERIOD)	1
DELTA ONE:	(EST NO. UNITS REQUIRED NEXT 10 DAYS)	1, 7
DELTA TWO:	(EST NO. UNITS BY ABO/RH NEXT 10 DAYS)	1, 3, 7
DELTA THREE:	(DESIRED DELIVERY DATE)	1
DELTA FOUR:	(DESIRED DELIVERY DESTINATION)	1, 4, 5
DELTA FIVE:	(RECEIVING OFFICIAL AT DESTINATION)	1, 5

NOTES:

1. OMIT LINES NOT APPLICABLE.

2. REPORT PERIOD IS AS OF 2400 LOCAL.

3. IF THE BRAVO AND DELTA LINES NEED TO BE USED MORE THAN ONCE TO REPORT DIFFERENT NUMBERS OF UNITS, GROUPS, TYPES, ETC., INFORMATION WILL BE REPORTED BY SEPARATING WITH A "/."

    EXAMPLE: BRAVO ONE: 10/20/30
                           BRAVO TWO: A+/B+/O+
                           BRAVO THREE: 10JAN/11JAN/12JAN

THIS IS INTERPRETED AS: ON HAND 10 UNITS A+ EXP DATE 10 JAN/20 UNITS B+ EXP DATE 11 JAN/30 UNITS O+ EXP DATE 12 JAN.

4. REPORT DESIRED DELIVERY DESTINATION ONLY IF DIFFERENT FROM LINE ALPHA THREE.

Figure C-2. Blood Status Report/Request (Sheet 1 of 2)

BLOOD STATUS REPORT/REQUEST

NOTES (continued):

5. REPORT RECEIVING OFFICIAL ONLY IF OTHER THAN LABORATORY PERSONNEL.

6. REPORT UNIT LOCATION IN GRID COORDINATES WHEN POSSIBLE AND ONLY IF CHANGED FROM LAST REPORT.

7. NORMALLY, ESTIMATED REQUIREMENTS WILL BE FOR THE DAY FOLLOWING THE LAST DAY OF SUPPLY ON HAND AND ON ORDER. SUPPLY LEVELS WILL BE ANNOUNCED IN APPROPRIATE PLANS AND ORDERS.

Figure C-2. Blood Status Report/Request (Sheet 2 of 2)

C.7 MEDICAL CENSUS REPORT

MEDICAL CENSUS REPORT

FM: (UNIT)
TO: (CATF/CLF)

SUBJ: MEDICAL CENSUS REPORT FOR MEDICAL REGULATING OFFICER

ALPHA: (MEDICAL UNIT REPORTING) *SEE NOTES 1, 5

BRAVO: (LOCATION IF CHANGED)

CHARLIE: (DTG AT END OF REPORT PERIOD) *SEE NOTE 2

DELTA: (TOTAL OPERATING BEDS AT END OF REPORTING) *SEE NOTE 3
DELTA ONE: (ICU BEDS)
DELTA TWO: (INTERMEDIATE CARE BEDS)
DELTA THREE: (MINIMAL CARE BEDS)

ECHO: (TOTAL PATIENTS ADMITTED DURING PERIOD AND BY SERVICE/CIVILIAN/POW) *SEE NOTE 4

FOXTROT: (TOTAL BEDS UNOCCUPIED AT END OF PERIOD)
FOXTROT ONE: (ICU BEDS UNOCCUPIED)
FOXTROT TWO: (INTERMEDIATE CARE BEDS UNOCCUPIED)
FOXTROT THREE: (MINIMAL CARE BEDS UNOCCUPIED)

GOLF: (TOTAL PATIENTS REMAINING AT END OF PERIOD BY SERVICE/CIVILIAN/POW) *SEE NOTE 4

HOTEL: (TOTAL PATIENTS RETURNED TO DUTY DURING PERIOD)

INDIA: (TOTAL PATIENTS EVACUATED DURING PERIOD)

JULIET: (TOTAL DEATHS IN FACILITIES DURING PERIOD BY SERVICE/CIVILIAN/POW) *SEE NOTE 4

KILO: (PATIENTS REQUIRING EVACUATION) *SEE NOTE 4
KILO ONE: (PATIENTS READY FOR EVAC NOT PREVIOUSLY REPORTED)
KILO TWO: (PATIENTS READY FOR EVAC PREVIOUSLY REPORTED BUT NOT EVACUATED)

LIMA: (UNUSUAL INCIDENCE OR OCCURRENCE OF DISEASE OR INJURY)

MIKE: (TOTAL OUTPATIENT VISITS DURING PERIOD)

NOVEMBER: (UNRESOLVED MEDICAL LOGISTICAL PROBLEMS)

NOTES:

1. SUBMITTED INITIALLY BY EVERY MTF WHEN IT BECOMES OPERATIONAL.

2. SUBSEQUENTLY, ALL MTFs MUST SUBMIT REPORT DAILY AT 0500.

Figure C-3. Medical Census Report (Sheet 1 of 2)

MEDICAL CENSUS REPORT

NOTES (continued):

3. WHEN REPORTING DELTA LINES, REPORT ONLY THOSE BEDS SET UP AND READY TO RECEIVE PATIENTS.

4. SUBMIT ONLY THOSE LINES REFLECTING A CHANGE FROM THE PREVIOUS REPORT.

5. SUBMITTED IN ADDITION TO THE SPOT STATUS REPORT.

Figure C-3. Medical Census Report (Sheet 2 of 2)

C.8 NINE-LINE EVACUATION REQUEST

LINE ITEM	FORMAT	SOURCE	NORMAL SOURCE	REASON
1. Location of pickup site	Encrypt the grid coordinates of the pickup site. When using the DRYAD Numeral Cipher, the same "SET" line will be used to encrypt the grid zone letters and the coordinates. To preclude misunderstanding, a statement is made that grid zone letters are included in the message (unless unit SOP specifies its use at all times).	From map	Unit leader(s)	To provide required patient pickup coordinates. To allow coordinating unit to plan route in the event of multiple patient pickups.
2. Radio frequency call sign, and button	Encrypt the frequency of the radio at the pickup site, not a relay frequency. The call sign, and suffix if used, of the pickup site POC may be transmitted in the clear.	From signal operation instruction	Radio telephone operator	To provide means of communication between evacuation vehicle and requesting unit while en route (e.g., obtain additional information or change in situation or directions).
3. Number of patients by precedence	Report only applicable information and encrypt the brevity codes: A — URGENT B — URGENT-SURG C — PRIORITY D — ROUTINE E — CONVENIENCE. If two or more categories must be reported in the same request, insert the word BREAK between each category.	From evaluation of patient(s)	Medic or senior person present	To assist in prioritizing missions by unit controlling the evacuation vehicles.
4. Special equipment required	Encrypt the applicable brevity codes: A — None B — Hoist C — Extraction equipment D — Ventilator.	From evaluation of patient or situation	Medic or senior person present	To ensure proper equipment is on board the evacuation vehicle prior to the start of the mission.

Figure C-4. Description of Medical Evacuation Request Preparation (Sheet 1 of 3)

LINE ITEM	FORMAT	SOURCE	NORMAL SOURCE	REASON
5. Number of patients by type	Report only applicable information and encrypt the brevity code: L+# of Pn — Litter A+# of Pnt — Ambulatory (sitting) If requesting MEDEVAC for both types, insert the word BREAK between the litter entry and the ambulatory entry.	From evaluation of patient(s)	Medic or senior person present	To ensure the appropriate number of evacuation vehicles are dispatched to the pickup site and are configured to carry the patients requiring evacuation.
6. (Wartime) Security of pickup site	Encrypt the brevity codes: N — No enemy troops in area P — Possible enemy troops in area (approach with caution) E — Enemy troops in area (approach with caution) X — Enemy troops in area (armed escort required).	From evaluation of the situation	Unit leader	To assist the evacuation crew in assessing the situation and to provide definitive guidance to the evacuation vehicle while en route (e.g., specific location of enemy for aircraft planning approach).
6. (Peacetime) Number and type of wound, injury, or illness	Specific information regarding patient wounds by type (gunshot or shrapnel). Report serious bleeding and patient blood type, if known.	From evaluation of patient	Medic or senior person present	To assist evacuation personnel in determining treatment and special equipment required.
7. Method of marking pickup site	Encrypt the brevity codes: A — Panels B — Pyrotechnic signal C — Smoke signal D — None E — Other.	Based on situation and availability of materiel	Medic or senior person present	To assist the evacuation crew in identifying the pickup location. Do not transmit the color of panels or smoke until the evacuation vehicle contacts the unit prior to its arrival. For security, the crew identifies the color and the unit verifies it.
8. Patient nationality and status	The number of patients in each category need not be transmitted. Encrypt only the applicable brevity codes: A — US military B — US civilian C — Non-US military D — Non-US civilian E — Enemy POW.	From evaluation of patient	Medic or senior person present	To assist in planning for destination facilities security. Ensure that an English-speaking representative is present at the pickup site.

Figure C-4. Description of Medical Evacuation Request Preparation (Sheet 2 of 3)

LINE ITEM	FORMAT	SOURCE	NORMAL SOURCE	REASON
9. (Wartime) Nuclear, biological, or chemical contamiation	Include this line only when applicable. Encrypt the applicable brevity codes: N — Nuclear B — Biological C — Chemical.	From situation	Medic or senior person present	To assist in planning the mission (e.g., type of evacuation vehicle, date, time).
9. (Peacetime) Terrain description	Include details of terrain features in and around proposed landing site. If possible, describe relationship of site to prominent terrain features (e.g., lake, mountain, tower).	From area survey	Personnel at site	To allow evacuation personnel to assess route/avenue of approach into area, especially if hoist operation is required.

Figure C-4. Description of Medical Evacuation Request Preparation (Sheet 3 of 3)

APPENDIX D

Examples of Status Boards Used in Medical Regulating

Four status boards are used in the medical regulating process: the Facilities Spot Status Board; the Blood Status Board; the consolidated Joining Report Board; and the Medical Regulating Status Board. (See Figures D-1 through D-4.) These boards provide the medical regulator and other HSS staff personnel with the capability to view current medical regulating issues and their statuses at a glance. Traditionally status boards have been constructed of thermoplastic mounting on a sheet of 1/2-inch plywood. Current status boards are developed using Excel® spreadsheets.

Data is recorded using a grease pencil or erasable marking pen. Regulators can make copies of the status board templates contained in this appendix to develop a running log of events throughout the entire operation. Regulators record information on the status boards and appropriate changes as they occur. The changes are then stored in a binder.

Note

Facilities will report their status every 24 hours, at a minimum. During periods of increased operations, report status more frequently but no less than every 6 hours.

FACILITY STATUS AS OF _____ (TIME AND DATE)										
UNIT CALL SIGN										
A. Operating Beds										
B. Beds Occupied										
C. Major OR										
OR Backlog — Patients										
OR Backlog — Hours of Surgery										
D. Minor OR										
OR Backlog — Patients										
OR Backlog — Hours of Surgery										
E. Patients Ready for Evacuation										
F. Patients Evacuated Out of the Operational Area										
G. Remarks										

Figure D-1. Facilities Spot Status Board Example

ACTUAL BLOOD STATUS AS OF _____ (TIME AND DATE)										
REPORTING UNIT										
A-Positive										
A-Negative										
B-Positive										
B-Negative										
O-Positive										
O-Negative										
AB-Positive										
AB-Negative										
Number of Walking Blood Donors (ABO/Rh Types)										
Refrigerators										
TOTAL UNITS										

Figure D-2. Blood Status Board Example

JOINING REPORT STATUS AS OF _____ (TIME AND DATE)										
REPORTING UNIT										
1. Number of Dedicated ORs										
2. Number of Other (Minor) ORs										
3. Number of Fixed x-ray Units										
4. Number of Portable x-ray Units										
5. Number of Blood Units on Hand										
6. Number of Blood Refrigerators and Capacity										
7. Number of Walking Blood Donors on Hand										
8. Number of Intensive Care Beds										
9. Number of Other Sickbay Beds										
10. Number of Overflow Beds										
11. Number of Medical Officers/Dental Officers/Physician Assistants (by Navy Officer Billet Classification (NOBC))										
12. Number of Hospital Corpsmen (by Navy Enlisted Classification (NEC))										
13. Number of Embarked/Augmented HSS Personnel (by Unit/Corps/NOBC/NEC)										

Figure D-3. Joining Report Board Example

Note

Create enough boxes to contain the required patient diagnostic codes specified in the OPLAN.

MEDICAL REGULATING STATUS AS OF _____ (TIME AND DATE)

HSS FACILITY	BEDS/BEDS OCCUPIED	(SEE NOTE)	(SEE NOTE)	(SEE NOTE)	(SEE NOTE)	(SEE NOTE)	(SEE NOTE)	ACTIVE REQUESTS FOR PATIENT MOVEMENT URGENT/PRIORITY/ROUTINE
	/							/ /
	/							/ /
	/							/ /
	/							/ /
	/							/ /
MASF/ASF	/							/ /
Returned to Duty								REMARKS/NOTES
Died of Wounds								
Intratheater Evacuations								
Intertheater Evacuations								
TOTALS								As of 0001 _____ (Date)

Figure D-4. Medical Regulating Status Board Example

APPENDIX E

Casualty Categorization and Prioritization

E.1 EVACUATION PRECEDENCE

Assignment of patient evacuation precedence is made by the senior military person present. This decision is based on the advice of the senior medical person at the scene, the patient's condition, and the tactical situation. Evacuation precedence provides the supporting medical unit and controlling HQ with information used in determining priorities for committing their evacuation assets. For this reason, correct assignment of evacuation precedence cannot be overemphasized.

Patients are evacuated as soon as possible, consistent with available resources and pending missions. Figure E-1 lists the categories of precedence and the criteria used in their assignment. Figure E-2 lists the evacuation categories and approximate evacuation time periods.

PRIORITY	PRECEDENCE	CRITERIA
I	Urgent	Patients that *require emergency, short-notice evacuation within a maximum of two hours:* to save life, limb, and eyesight to prevent serious complications of the injury, serious illness, or permanent disability.
IA	Urgent-Surgical	Patients that *require far forward surgical intervention:* to save life to stabilize for further evacuation.
II	Priority	Patients that *require prompt medical care within a maximum of four hours:* to prevent the medical condition from deteriorating to an urgent precedence, to prevent unnecessary pain or disability, to provide required treatment not available locally.
III	Routine	Patients who *do not require immediate medical attention* and whose condition is not expected to deteriorate significantly. *Evacuation should be made within 24 hours.*
IV	Convenience	Patients for whom *evacuation* by medical vehicle *is a matter of medical convenience rather than necessity.*

Figure E-1. Priority Levels and Criteria for Evacuation Precedence

CATEGORY	ARMY	NAVY	MARINE CORPS	AIR FORCE
Urgent	Within 2 Hours	Within 2 Hours	Within 2 Hours	As Soon As Possible
Priority	Within 4 Hours	Within 4 Hours	Within 4 Hours	Within 24 Hours
Routine	Within 24 Hours	Within 24 Hours	Within 24 Hours	Within 72 Hours

Figure E-2. Evacuation Time Periods

Note

The categories of evacuation precedence are urgent, priority, and routine. The evacuation time periods are flexible, mission dependent, and vary greatly among the types of evacuation assets used by the Services.

E.2 TRIAGE

Triage is the categorization of casualties for the priority of treatment and evacuation. It is one of the most important tasks in casualty care, requiring the most informed judgment, knowledge, and courage. Triage is a continuing process. The individual assigned should be the most capable and experienced health care provider available.

E.2.1 Principles of Triage

The following are principles of triage:

1. Accomplish the greatest good for the greatest number of casualties.

2. Employ the most efficient use of available resources.

3. Return personnel to duty as soon as possible.

E.2.1.1 Triage Factors

The following are triage factors:

1. Number of casualties requiring treatment.

2. Medical resources available to treat casualties (to include personnel and equipment).

3. Attention toward easily treated conditions.

   a. Rapid and accurate assessments.

   b. Continuous reassessment and retriage of all casualties.

E.2.1.2 Categories of Casualty Triage

The first formal triage establishes the patient's category. These categories are color coded and are recognized as follows:

1. Category I. Immediate (Red Tag). This category includes all compromises to a patient's ABCs. If immediate medical attention is not provided, the patient will die. These medical procedures should not be time consuming and should concern only those casualties with high chance of survival. Examples include:

   a. Airway compromise. Performing an emergency cricothyroidotomy for an obstructed airway

   b. Breathing compromise. Performing a needle thoracentesis to decompress a tension pneumothorax

   c. Circulation compromise. Applying a tourniquet to an arterial bleed.

2. Category II. Delayed (Yellow Tag). This category includes any injury that may be serious and potentially life threatening. The patient may require extensive and intensive treatment but is not expected to significantly deteriorate over several hours. Patients in this category can safely wait until Category I patients have been stabilized. Examples include:

   a. Compensated shock

   b. Fractures, dislocations, or injuries causing circulatory compromise

   c. Severe bleeding controlled with a tourniquet or other means

   d. Open fractures and dislocations

   e. Abdominal, thoracic, spinal, or head injuries

   f. Uncomplicated major burns.

3. Category III. Minimal (Green Tag). This category, also called the walking wounded, includes patients with injuries that require treatment but are unlikely to deteriorate over the next few days. These individuals have relatively minor injuries and can effectively care for themselves or can be helped by untrained personnel. Examples include:

   a. Minor lacerations

   b. Abrasions

   c. Fractures of small bones

   d. Minor burns and strains.

4. Category IV. Expectant (Black Tag). This category is comprised of patients whose treatment would be time consuming and extremely complicated coupled with a low chance of survival. The extent of their treatment depends on available supplies and manpower. These patients should not be abandoned; every effort should be devoted to their comfort. Once all immediate and delayed patients are treated, expectant patients are retriaged and treated based on remaining medical supplies and personnel. Examples include:

   a. Cardiac arrest from any cause

   b. Massive brain/head trauma

   c. Second- or third-degree burns over 70 percent of body surface area

   d. Massive exposure to radiation.

E.2.2 Treatment Priorities

After the first and formal triage, Category I, Immediate (Red Tag), patients are further triaged into treatment priorities. The most severely injured immediate patients are treated first.

E.2.2.1 First Priority

The first-priority casualties suffer from one or more of the following conditions:

1. Asphyxia

2. Respiratory obstruction from mechanical causes

3. Open/tension pneumothorax

4. Maxillofacial wounds

5. Shock due to major external hemorrhage

6. Major hemorrhage

7. Visceral (abdominal) injuries

8. Cardio/pericardial injuries

9. Massive muscle damage

10. Major fractures

11. Multiple wounds

12. Severe burns over 20 percent of body surface area.

E.2.2.2 Second Priority

The second-priority casualties suffer from one or more of the following conditions:

1. Visceral (abdominal) injuries with perforations of the intestinal tract, wounds of the genitourinary tract, or thoracic wounds without asphyxia

2. Vascular injuries needing repair

3. Closed cerebral injuries with increasing levels of consciousness

4. Burns under 20 percent of body surface area involving face, hands, feet, and genitalia.

E.2.2.3 Third Priority

The third-priority casualties suffer from one or more of the following conditions:

1. Soft-tissue wounds without major muscle damage

2. Minor fractures and dislocations

3. Injuries of the eye

4. Maxillofacial injuries without asphyxia

5. Burns under 20 percent of body surface area.

APPENDIX F

Afloat and Shipboard Medical Evacuation Checklists

F.1 AFLOAT MEDICAL EVACUATION CHECKLIST

Date/Time Initiated:		
Rank:	Full Name:	
Patient SSN:	Patient Command/Unit:	
Date/Time Completed:		
Patient Diagnosis (IDC-9):		
Patient Classification:		
Patient Status: (Circle One)		
Stable	Conscious	Unconscious
Ambulatory		Stretcher
Medical Attendant	Nonmedical Attendant	Guard Required
Attending Medical Officer (Name):		
Contact gaining accepting MTF MO (Use Flag Plot POTS):		
Accepting Physician Information:		
Narrative Summary (Write Legibly):		

Figure F-1. Afloat Medical Evacuation Checklist (Sheet 1 of 2)

	Discharge orders, en route orders, and prescriptions						
	Prepare to talk with NOK; NOK information						
Nurse (Name):							
	Patient is ready to leave per NTTP 4-02.2M, Navy appendices						
	Patient records and baggage tags prepared						
Records Checklist:							
	Funded TAD Orders		Service Record		Pay Advance		Medical Record
	Dental Record		Narrative Summary		Consult		Labs/x rays
	Inpatient Record Copy				Valuables		
	Fill prescriptions						
	Uniform, civilian clothes, identification card, passport, and toiletries accompany the patient						
SMDR/MRCO (Name):							
	Notify chain of command and medical authority						
	Debrief; include blue and green side administrative and disbursing personnel						
	Arrange for orders through personnel						
	Make flight arrangements with HDC						
	Pick up checks or advances from Disbursing						
	Prepare MEDEVAC MSG within 24 hours of MEDEVAC						
	Enter information into database						
	Start patient tracking						

Figure F-1. Afloat Medical Evacuation Checklist (Sheet 2 of 2)

F.2 SHIPBOARD TREATMENT/EVACUATION TEAM CHECKLIST

TASK DESCRIPTION	VERIFIED
Approval to MEDEVAC (SMO/SMDR)	
1. Recommendation/concurrence to MEDEVAC from provider, CSG/ESG/ATF surgeon, SMDR, and accepting physician (afloat or ashore, civilian or military).	
2. Permission to MEDEVAC from AOR patient movement center.	
3. Agreement to MEDEVAC from TGRO (if using contractor provider network).	
4. Permission to MEDEVAC obtained from the patient's COC.	
5. Recommendation to evacuate obtained from the provider's COC.	
Administrative Issues. Administrative Officer and Patient's COC	
1. Funded orders for a period of 30 days for patient and attendant/escort (consider cash advancement) (Administrative Officer).	
2. Proper attire (civilian and military) (COC).	
3. Personal items (shaving gear, dental paste, toothbrush, etc.) (COC).	
4. Patient identification (military identification card and/or passport if available).	
5. Patient luggage (maximum two pieces: seabag less than 70 lbs. and a carry-on).	
Air Operations, Supply, Communication(s) Officers (AIR OPS/SUPPO/COMMO)	
1. Send naval message (drafted by the medical provider) to MEDEVAC and/or ask for assistance and/or notify numbered fleet and nearest MTF (COMMO).	
2. Provide e-mail/chat capabilities to provider (SIPRNET/NIPRNET) if naval message is not indicated (COMMO).	
3. Provide telephone capabilities as necessary (COMMO).	
4. Set up air and/or ship-to-ship and/or boat evacuation (AIR OPS).	
5. Set up ground transportation if ship is in port or medical for local ambulance (SUPPO).	
Notification and Patient Tracking (SMDR/MRCO/XO)	
1. Notify numbered fleet surgeon (naval message/e-mail/telephone) (SMDR/MRCO).	
2. Notify ISIC medical (SMDR/MRCO).	
3. Notify nearest MTF (naval message/e-mail/telephone) (SMDR/MRCO).	
4. Notify fleet liaison of receiving or closest MTF (naval message/e-mail/telephone) (SMDR/MRCO).	
5. Notify U.S. Embassy Defense Attaché Office if patient remains hospitalized in the HN (naval message/e-mail/telephone) (SMDR/MRCO).	
6. Notify husbanding agent medical representative of HN, if in port. Medical representative will assist in arranging care, reports, and medical payment of services rendered (SMDR/MRCO).	

Figure F-2. Shipboard Treatment/Evacuation Team Checklist (Sheet 1 of 2)

TASK DESCRIPTION	VERIFIED
7. Notify NOK, if indicated (XO/Command Master Chief or Senior Marine Corps Unit Rep). If possible, allow patient to speak with NOK.	
8. Notify SMO/accepting physician/hospital/clinic (SMDR/MRCO).	
9. Initiate patient tracking (SMDR/MRCO).	
10. Send situation report and safety message to appropriate agencies, if indicated (SMDR/XO).	
Brief the Patient and/or Escort (SMDR/SMO)	
1. Where is the patient going? Specify installation/command.	
2. To whom does the patient report? Specify person's name.	
3. What is/are the patient's restriction(s)? Diet, ambulatory, litter, 24/7 watch (if psych).	
4. Enough medication for travel period? Recommend 7–10 days.	
5. Enough medical supplies available for travel period?	
6. Latest documentation of current medical problems, including medical/dental, labs, x rays, physician orders, international certificate of vaccinations, etc.? Give to patient or escort.	
7. List POCs. Ship, hospital, MTF, physician, and fleet liaison names and numbers given to patient or escort.	
8. Provide name and number of patient's emergency contact, if available. Normally, ISIC medical POC.	
9. Provide a full itinerary with final and all known intermediate destinations.	
10. Write all of above information and include in records to be given to patient/escort.	
Equipment (Medical Team)	
1. Verify supplies needed for the patient (dressings, bandages, etc.).	
2. Verify all equipment is fully operational, if required.	
3. Label all equipment with the ship's name and address. (Easier to claim at completion of MEDEVAC.)	

Figure F-2. Shipboard Treatment/Evacuation Team Checklist (Sheet 2 of 2)

REFERENCES

The development of NTTP 4-02.2M/MCRP 4-11.1G (MAY 2007) is based upon the following sources.

AJP 4-10, Allied Joint Medical Support Doctrine.

CJCSM 3500.03 (series), Joint Training Manual for the Armed Forces of the United States.

CJCSM 3500.04 (series), Universal Joint Task List (UJTL).

COMNAVSURFORINST 6000.1, Shipboard Medical Procedures Manual.

COMNAVWARDEVCOM, TACMEMO 3-07.7-06, Domestic Disaster Relief Operation Planning.

U.S. Department of Homeland Security (DHS), National Response Plan.
   Emergency Support Function Annexes.
      Emergency Support Function #1, Transportation Annex.
      Emergency Support Function #8, Public Health and Medical Services Annex.

FM 8-55, Planning for Health Service Support.

JP 1-02, Department of Defense Dictionary of Military and Associated Terms.

JP 3-0, Joint Operations.

JP 4-02, Health Service Support.

JP 5-0, Joint Operation Planning.

MCRP 4-11.1E, Health Service Support Field Reference Guide (draft).

MCRP 5-12D, Organization of Marine Corps Forces.

MCWP 3-11.4, Helicopterborne Operations.

MCWP 4-11.1, Health Service Support Operations.

MCWP 5-1, Marine Corps Planning Process.

MSTP Pamphlet 5-0.3, MAGTF Planner's Reference Manual.

NTRP 1-02, Navy Supplement to the DOD Dictionary of Military and Associated Terms.

NTTP 3-02.1M/MCWP 3-31.5, Ship-to-Shore Movement.

NWP 4-02, Naval Expeditionary Health Service Support Afloat and Ashore.

NWP 5-01, Navy Planning.

OPNAVINST 3500.38/MCO 3500.26/USCG COMDTINST 3500.1 (series), Universal Naval Task List (UNTL).

OPNAVINST 3501 (series), Projected Operational Environment (POE) and Required Operational Capabilities (ROC).

STANAG 2931, Camouflage of the Red Cross and Red Crescent on Land in Tactical Operations.

LIST OF ACRONYMS AND ABBREVIATIONS

ACE	aviation combat element (MAGTF)
AE	aeromedical evacuation
AELT	aeromedical evacuation liaison team
AES	aeromedical evacuation system
AIR OPS	air operations officer
AJP	Allied Joint Publication
ALO	air liaison officer
AOA	amphibious objective area
AOR	area of responsibility
AS	submarine tender
ASE	air support element
ATF	amphibious task force
AXP	ambulance exchange point
BAS	battalion aid station
BES	beach evacuation station
BLT	battalion landing team
BUMED	Bureau of Medicine and Surgery
C2	command and control
CASEVAC	casualty evacuation
CATF	commander, amphibious task force
CBRN	chemical, biological, radiological, or nuclear
CC	command center
CCDR	combatant commander
CE	combat element (MAGTF)

CIC	combat information center
CICWO	combat information center watch officer
CJCSM	Chairman of the Joint Chiefs of Staff manual
CLB	combat logistics battalion
CLC	combat logistics company
CLF	commander, landing force
CO	commanding officer
COC	chain of command
COCOM	combatant command (command authority)
COMMO	communication(s) officer
COMNAVSURFORINST	Commander, Naval Surface Forces instruction
CONUS	continental United States
CRTS	casualty receiving and treatment ship
CSG	carrier strike group
CSSOC	combat service support operations center
CV/CVN	aircraft carrier/aircraft carrier, nuclear
DASC	direct air support center
DHHS	Department of Health and Human Services
DHS	Department of Homeland Security
DOD	Department of Defense
DS	direct support
DTG	date-time group
EMF	expeditionary medical facility
ESF	emergency support function
ESG	expeditionary strike group
°F	degrees Fahrenheit
FM	field manual (Army)

FRC	forward resuscitative care
FRSS	forward resuscitative surgery system
FST	fleet surgical team
FWD	forward
GCE	ground combat element (MAGTF)
GPMRC	Global Patient Movement Requirements Center
GS	general support
H&S	headquarters and service
HAC	helicopter aircraft commander
HDC	helicopter direction center
HES	helicopter evacuation station
HHQ	higher headquarters
HMMWV	high mobility multipurpose wheeled vehicle
HN	host nation
HQ	headquarters
HSAP	Health Services Augmentation Program
HSC	helicopter support center
HSS	health service support
HSSE	health service support element
HSSO	health service support officer
HST	helicopter support team
IDC	independent duty corpsman
ISIC	immediate superior-in-command
ITV	in-transit visibility
JFLCC	joint force land component commander
JP	joint publication
JPMRC	joint patient movement requirements center

J/TPMRC	joint/theater patient movement requirements center
LCE	logistics combat element (MAGTF)
LF	landing force
LFSP	landing force support party
LHA	amphibious assault ship (general purpose)
LHD	amphibious assault ship (multipurpose)
LMCC	logistic and movement control center
LPD	amphibious transport dock
LPO	leading petty officer
LSD	landing ship dock
LZ	landing zone
MAG	Marine aircraft group
MAGTF	Marine air-ground task force
MAO	medical administrative officer
MARDIV	Marine division
MASF	mobile aeromedical staging facility
MAW	Marine aircraft wing
MCA	movement control agency
MCRP	Marine Corps reference publication
MCT	Marine Corps Task
MCTL	Marine Corps Task List
MCWP	Marine Corps warfighting publication
MEB	Marine expeditionary brigade
MEDEVAC	medical evacuation
MEDREGNET	medical regulating network
MEF	Marine expeditionary force
METT-T	mission, enemy, terrain and weather, troops and support available—time available

MEU	Marine expeditionary unit
MIACG	Medical Interagency Coordination Group
MLG	Marine logistics group
MOUT	military operations on urbanized terrain
MRCO	medical regulating control officer
MRT	medical regulating team
MSC	Medical Service Corps
MSOC	medical support operations center
MSTP	Marine Air-Ground Task Force (MAGTF) Staff Training Program
MTF	medical treatment facility
MWSG	Marine wing support group
MWSS	Marine wing support squadron
NATO	North Atlantic Treaty Organization
NAVFAC	Naval Facilities Engineering Command
NAVFOR	Navy forces
NAVSUP	Naval Supply Systems Command
NDMS	National Disaster Medical System
NECC	Navy Expeditionary Combat Command
NIPRNET	Non-Secure Internet Protocol Router Network
NOK	next of kin
NRP	National Response Plan
NTTL	Navy Tactical Task List
NTTP	Navy tactics, techniques, and procedures
NWP	Navy warfare publication
OCONUS	outside the continental United States
OIC	officer in charge
OPCON	operational control

OPLAN	operation plan
OPNAVINST	Chief of Naval Operations instruction
OPORD	operation order
PCS	primary control ship
PEO	patient evacuation officer
PET	patient evacuation team
PMI	patient movement item
PMR	patient movement request
PMRC	patient movement requirements center
POC	point of contact
PZ	pickup zone
RAS	regimental aid station
RLT	regimental landing team
ROMO	range of military operations
SCS	secondary control ship
SIPRNET	SECRET Internet Protocol Router Network
SMDR	senior medical department representative
SMO	senior medical officer
SOP	standard operating procedure
STANAG	standardization agreement (NATO)
STP	shock trauma platoon
SUPPO	supply officer
TACC	tanker airlift control center
TACMEMO	tactical memorandum
T-AH	hospital ship
TAO	tactical action officer
TAR/HR	tactical air request/helicopter request

TF	task force
TGRO	TRICARE Global Remote Overseas
TPMRC	theater patient movement requirements center
TTP	tactics, techniques, and procedures
UJTL	Universal Joint Task List
UNTL	Universal Naval Task List
USA	United States Army
USAF	United States Air Force
USCG	United States Coast Guard
USMC	United States Marine Corps
USN	United States Navy
USNORTHCOM	United States Northern Command
USTRANSCOM	United States Transportation Command
VS	visual signal
XO	executive officer

LIST OF EFFECTIVE PAGES

Effective Pages	Page Numbers
MAY 2007	1 thru 20
MAY 2007	1-1 thru 1-6
MAY 2007	2-1 thru 2-4
MAY 2007	3-1 thru 3-8
MAY 2007	4-1 thru 4-12
MAY 2007	5-1 thru 5-20
MAY 2007	A-1, A-2
MAY 2007	B-1 thru B-14
MAY 2007	C-1 thru C-14
MAY 2007	D-1 thru D-6
MAY 2007	E-1 thru E-6
MAY 2007	F-1 thru F-4
MAY 2007	Reference-1, Reference-2
MAY 2007	LOAA-1 thru LOAA-8
MAY 2007	LEP-1, LEP-2